LOSE WEIGHT
&
FEEL GREAT:

Transform Yourself
the Total Body Way

Billy Hofacker, B.S., CSCS

Limits of Liability and Disclaimer of Warranty

Warning – Disclaimer

ISBN-13: 978-1547276806
ISBN-10: 1547276800

ACKNOWLEDGMENTS

TO SAY THIS book was written by me, Billy Hofacker, would be an understatement. Without the contributions made by the following people, this book wouldn't exist.

I'd like to thank my many mentors and coaches over the years. Specifically, I'd like to acknowledge my current coaches. Pat Rigsby, you continue to push me to become better, not just as a businessman but as a person. I also thank my business coaches at EntreLeadership for the time, knowledge, and care invested in me. Being an Entre-Leader, someone who leads a cause or venture to grow and prosper, is one of my proudest titles.

In addition, I would like to thank my writing coach, Donna Kozik—Donna, you are everything I hope to be in a coach. You motivate and inspire me, guide me, and hold me accountable. I'm a better writer and speaker because of you.

I feel indebted to my friends and team at Total Body Boot Camp and Performance Center (TBBC) —Bill Riccio, Sam Gilchrist, Kathy Conlon, Bill Powers, Lori Carty, and KC Reilly—for their passion and support. Working with you every day is one of my greatest blessings.

And I want to make a special acknowledgement of our clients at Total Body Boot Camp and Performance Center. We call them Warriors. You blow me away every time I see your dedication to your health and fitness and to TBBC. I hope to be able to inspire you as much as you have me.

Special thanks to my most important team—the one at home!

My girls: Alyssa, I'm so proud of the young lady you're becoming, and Olivia, you are such a joy to our family and to this world.

My wife, Melissa, you are committed wholeheartedly to our family. For that and for so many other reasons I am eternally grateful for you. I love you with all that I am.

Finally, and above all else, to my heavenly Father—Your grace wins every time.

WHAT PEOPLE ARE SAYING ABOUT BILLY HOFACKER

He Keeps Me Motivated

"Billy makes you feel comfortable during every session and you feel like you're part of a family. Even when the workout is tough, he keeps pushing me to do my best and has a unique way of keeping me motivated."

– Cathy Fay

Pushes You to Be Better

"As soon as I met Billy, I could tell he didn't look at people as customers. He cares about the individual and takes pride in helping them reach their goals. I look forward to all of his training sessions as he pushes you to be better physically and mentally."

– Salvatore Pugliese

Lost Over Fifty Pounds

"Billy has proved to be an amazing motivator and so knowledgeable that when I listened to his advice, I lost over 50 pounds and gained strength I never thought was possible. He has the ability to see possibilities and strengths in people that they do not always see in themselves and helps them to reach goals they never thought they could!

"He genuinely wants to show people how to be happy with their lives and how with a positive attitude your view of the world can change! Billy's compassion and empathy for others is immeasurable. Billy is a man of character, a man who believes in friendship, who understands the commitment to family, to honesty, and who will build you up, will encourage you to do better, be better. I have seen the impact he has made in so many lives and I am very, very proud to know him!"

– Sam Gilchrist

Walked Through It All With Me

"When I first went to TBBC I was skeptical, but Billy Hofacker was so wonderful and truly cared about what I wanted to accomplish. He walked through it all with me. First training session was tough but he was so supportive and never pushed me too hard. He never made me feel like I was behind or couldn't do it. He is truly a wonderful coach! This is more than a job for William."

– Jaime Davino

Doesn't Matter Your Age or Physical Ability

"I have been an athlete my entire life, but as you get older it gets tougher and tougher to try to stay in shape. I'm 57 and it's very easy to blame the job or the commute or the expense as reasons to stop exercising. TBBC was my savior. It doesn't matter your age or physical ability. Billy has created an environment where people of all ages and abilities can take a class together. All come out of it feeling like they got a great workout but never like they had to try to keep up. I know I could try to do this at home on my own but many of us just need that little push. I applaud his system and would highly recommend this to anyone that needs that little push every day to do something for your health as well as physical and mental attitude."

– Barry Levine

Never Boring

"Billy is truly dedicated to your health and fitness. He has created a family environment and is always motivating and encouraging you do to more, to be better. He talks the talk and walks the walk. He would never tell you to do something he wouldn't be willing to do himself. He creates fun workouts, which you become addicted to. It is certainly never boring. He will push you past your limits, but only to make you stronger, make you healthier, make you better! Thanks Billy for being a trainer and friend!"

– Raquel Modica

Cares About People

"Billy Hofacker genuinely cares about people and their personal health journey. His motivational skills and positive attitude create an environment where everyone is on the same journey to being healthier, both physically and mentally. Thanks Billy!"

– Patty Werner

Kind and Encouraging

"Billy Hofacker has been so helpful with my weight loss endeavor. He does it in a kind and encouraging way while leading by example with his healthy and focused lifestyle."

– Bonnie Perlman

Great Motivator

"Billy is so encouraging and a great motivator. He cares about every one of his clients. All the trainers are great motivators also. I feel like TBBC is my second family."

– Nancy Harms

Vibrant Personality and Energy

"After hearing Billy Hofacker speak at a public event for Toastmasters, his passion for fitness and desire to do his work in the world was evident. I trusted my own instinct and connected with him to join TBBC. His vibrant personality and energy is displayed in his work. A great addition to the fitness field."

– Patricia Stones

Positive Energy and Guidance

"Billy's positive energy and guidance have helped me so much. He is a man who cares about people, his employees, and gives back by donating to great causes. Mostly what I admire is his positive motivation to his life, his family, and others. In short I see a great man and great things to come his way in the years to come. Thanks Billy for all you have done for me and others, to make all here at TBBC a family."

– Warren Hirt

Great Mentor and Motivator

"Billy has become a great mentor and motivator. He's always there to guide and help me, and seems to truly care about me as a person. He made me feel like a part of his family (the TBBC family). I joined many different gyms before, and somehow I never continued with them. I truly believe that the one reason why I have stayed with TBBC for over 2 years is because of Billy Hofacker and his team. They make you feel like you are always welcomed, and that you are home—it's a place where everyone knows your name, a place where everyone is glad you came, never mocking you for what you can and cannot do, always motivating and inspiring everyone who walks through the doors. Billy Hofacker is TBBC and I believe he cares deeply for his family and the whole 'TBBC family.' I am honored that I am part of his very special TBBC family. Thank you Billy for all that you do!"

– Patricia Stork

Humble and Inspiring

"Billy is first and foremost a humble and inspiring person. He is a person who lives his truth by leading by example. During my interview upon joining the TBBC FAMILY it was evident that Billy was not just about making a sale. He truly cares about making you feel part of the TBBC family. He has implemented this culture throughout the TBBC experience. He shares his pearls of wisdom freely and is a great source of inspiration and motivation. Thank you Billy for all you have done to make my transition process a great experience. TBBC IS LIFE!"

– Sonji Crawford-Clark

Example of Goal Achievement

"What I love about Billy Hofacker is that he absolutely walks the walk when it comes to motivation and self-improvement. He makes himself the example of growth and goal-achievement through hard work and perseverance, and then encourages everyone to join him."

– Clarice Joos

Best Decision Ever

"Working with Billy was the best decision ever. I've joined regular gyms so many times before, and after a few months I just stop going. After 3 months of going to TBBC I had lost just a few pounds and I was feeling discouraged. I received a newsletter you sent out about a member being stuck and all of a sudden she started losing weight when she was about to give up. That really motivated me. I told you how I appreciated that newsletter coming in the mail because it came at a perfect time for me. I managed to lose 35 pounds by March and I was feeling amazing. You are an excellent motivator that cares and appreciates his clients."

– Maria Jimenez

Energy That Is Contagious

"Billy Hofacker has an energy that is contagious. He is a motivator! Billy gets to know all of his clients and takes a personal interest in their journey. It is truly refreshing!"

– Janice Spicijaric

Thank Goodness for Smaller Belts

"I just wanted to thank you for your motivation, guidance, encouragement and support with the nutrition and fitness coaching. I have lost a total of 23 pounds, which I am sure is more because I have gained muscle from my training with you and I feel great.

"Most importantly I received my blood test results from my doctor and they came down so much in such a short period of time that my doctor said it was 'remarkable' how the numbers turned around for the positive.

"I could not have accomplished this without your encouragement and support.

"Thank you again and I blame you for not having any clothes that fit. Thank goodness for smaller belts."

– Andy Sherman

Gift to Inform, Instruct, and Motivate

"Billy Hofacker was a guest speaker for a program I run called First Place. Every week I have a different speaker share some aspect of health, including physical, spiritual, or emotional health issues. Billy's vast knowledge of the physical health field was a great addition to our program. Billy has a real gift to inform, instruct and to motivate those he is speaking with. My members very much enjoyed hearing Billy share and have requested we ask him back in the near future."

– Donna Kirkland

CONTENTS

MY STORY

PEOPLE ASK WHAT caused me to dedicate my life to fitness. Believe it or not, I haven't always been a picture of muscle and self-discipline. In fact, growing up I was skinny and not particularly strong. But, I had an older brother I had to defend myself against. My brother played a big part of my formative years, but it wasn't the warm Leave It to Beaver relationship. Far from it.

I'm the youngest of three. While I have many happy memories growing up and much to be thankful for, life wasn't always easy back then. For example, one time my brother took a bat to my head, leaving a baseball-sized lump.

Everyone has struggles in life. This was mine for many years.

Later, I became stronger because of it.

As I got older I started learning different ways to improve myself.

We all have problems in our lives. They help mold us and make us who we are. I don't regret a thing because my experiences shaped me and I believe God had a plan for my life and for my family all along.

As I got older I became determined to make something of myself. When I was in high school, I began lifting weights and really focusing on sports. Sports served as a great outlet. I was able to forget about my problems. It felt so good to have something I was good at and a part of. And I ran with it. In high school, I played basketball for my town league as well as my school team. Every spare minute I had was spent honing my skills. I eventually made it onto one of the best traveling high school teams in the country. My coach, Amir, served as a great mentor. He believed in me and started talking about all of my possibilities. He genuinely cared. He would talk to me about my grades, college, and even gave me advice on dating.

I didn't realize it at the time, but the bullying I experienced early in life served as fuel for my fire to get better and stronger. In the summer after high school, I got up before 5 a.m. to do drills at the park. While my friends were watching TV, I was doing push-ups, sit-ups, and jumping rope. I remember being in the gym Friday nights putting just a little more weight on the bar each week. As I struggled through the repetitions, I had a vision of becoming stronger. Every time I felt like giving up, I'd push just a little more.

Soon after high school, I discovered Brazilian Jiu-Jitsu (BJJ). BJJ is a sport and art that requires a tremendous amount of discipline and dedication. It helped me train my mind and my body and to push myself to my physical and mental limits. I received a black belt in BJJ after many years of training and won competitions at the highest level. I also began diving into personal training, and I found my passion in helping others be their strongest, fittest, best selves.

Since I was a young boy, I've grown in a lot of ways. I'm so thankful for where I am now emotionally and spiritually. I've learned to be content and I have overcome anxiety. I'm excited about each day and the opportunity it brings, the opportunity to move closer to fulfilling my potential. The difficulties I experienced caused me to seek God and He's done amazing things in my life. I'm active in my church and I have significance and a purpose now. This is the greatest gift. I met and married the kindest, sweetest, and most beautiful woman in the world, Melissa. We have two precious daughters, Alyssa and Olivia.

Professionally, I've been able to open two private training facilities where my team and I help busy people lose weight and live their lives to the fullest. My team and I are working hard each day to build something special. Based on the feedback we get from our members, we are making a real difference. You will hear many of those awesome stories throughout this book.

Helping my team grow and doing work that matters with them is deeply fulfilling. We are more of a family than a bunch of people who just work together. I have to pinch myself sometimes because although it's hard work it can feel too good to be true.

I have come so far. I feel that I lived through many obstacles that I was able to overcome. Now I have a great life and this is what I want for others, which is why I wrote this book. You're going to learn a lot. I want you to see good things in your life.

You might not have been beat up by a bully of a brother when you were growing up, but I bet you had your own struggles, whether they were in person or within. Part of the reason I'm writing this book is to show you that you can accomplish your goals, even if you think you have obstacles that are too great.

I believe in you.

ABOUT THIS BOOK

WHILE READING THIS book you may be surprised how little specific exercise information there is. This is intentional. After helping busy people lose weight for almost 20 years, my team and I have developed the most effective fat burning programs possible. And the programs are actually fun!

When it comes to losing weight, here are some things you should know…

- **No One Size Fits All Programs** – When new clients come into our facility we do what we call a Starting Point. Essentially, it's an assessment of where they are starting from. A baseline so we can develop a program and see their progress. Without this information it would make very little sense to provide a program. With that said, if you'd like to get an idea for the best plan for you, schedule a free "Success in Fitness" Strategy Session with us and we'll get you going in the right direction. We'll also make sure it's safe! You can do that by visiting www.lifitnessbootcamp.com.

- **Every Program Works** – Wait, this seems to counter the first point. The reality is they are both true. While there isn't one program that is ideal for everyone, any program (for the most part) can work. The best program is the one that is safe, fun, and that you actually do.

- **It's Not the Main Thing** – Believe it or not, it's not about the Xs and Os or push-ups and squats. This book goes much deeper. You can find exercise programs by doing a simple Google search. With this book I wanted to focus on the areas that hold most people back. While there is a ton of practical "do this" info, I will go into deeper issues such as mindset, habit change, and emotional factors.

Although there will be some specific weight loss tactics and tips, we will be looking at the bigger picture and going a bit deeper. It's more than a diet or recipe. I'll be sharing information on…

- Developing a success mindset

- How to become more consistent

- 10 ways to stop self-sabotaging yourself

- Juggling family and fitness

- Preventing boredom in your fitness routine

- The most important meal of the day

- A simple plan to make healthy food choices

- Beating procrastination

- Much more

The best part is it's all super simple. You can see fantastic results by implementing one small idea at a time. These mindset and lifestyle attitudes will help you with your weight loss goals and beyond, from the gym to all other aspects in your life.

I'm so excited to be on this journey together with you! The fitness and weight loss puzzle is more of a behavior change thing than a head knowledge thing. Let's get started!

CHAPTER 1:

MINDSET: HOW TO SET YOURSELF UP FOR SUCCESS

ONE OF THE biggest differences between successful people and their counterparts is their mindset. In this chapter, I'll explain how you can set yourself up for success by thinking BIG. You will also learn the proper way to set goals.

> *"Your attitude is either your best friend or your worst enemy, your greatest asset or your greatest liability."*
> – *John Maxwell*

I've been helping people transform their bodies and lives for a long time, almost 20 years. I've also worked with some of the most successful entrepreneurs and athletes on the planet. I don't say this to impress you. I say it to impress upon you that I have a unique perspective.

The reality is there isn't much difference between the wildly successful people and those whom success eludes. I started with this chapter for a reason. I want to explain some of the small steps you can make regarding mindset that could make all the difference for you. While you may want to get right to the "fat loss tricks," I know that whatever information I provide to you will be of little value if you don't have a solid foundation. You wouldn't set out to build a house and start with the roof, would you? Trust me on this.

I love the Maxwell quote at the start of this section about your attitude being your best friend or your worst enemy. I've seen it in action. In fact, we have it painted on the wall at our facility. Since I've been working with so many people (well into the thousands) for so long, I can often tell how someone will do just based on their attitude. I've been surprised before, but I can often gauge someone's attitude by the words they use. For example, if they say something like, "I'm fat. I always quit. Nothing works," then I know we have our work cut out. It's no surprise that this individual needs to do some re-phrasing since words are so powerful. This next example might surprise you. When someone says something like, "You watch. I'm gonna be your best success story ever," I cringe. The reason I cringe is…

Actions speak louder than words. This is important to keep in mind as you set yourself up for success on your fitness journey. Behavioral change is not easy (more on that later). The person who starts off bragging has some heavy lifting to do, and they haven't even started yet. Oftentimes, they've had some extremely negative habits for decades. When they minimize that reality they are setting themselves up for failure. Our biggest success stories over the years didn't say much. They listened to us and followed through. They showed up consistently, put their heads down, and charged forward. They made small changes over time.

The Greatest Obstacle to Success: Self Doubt

Meet Donna! Check out an e-mail Donna sent us after her experience on the program…

> "Since joining TBBC, I've lost 7 pounds. I know it's not a lot, but what I've gained is a lot more: I feel stronger, more positive, and ready to make a change. Thanks to all the trainers for being patient with me. When I started TBBC, I knew I needed to do something about my weight, but I didn't really believe in

myself at the time. Now, I'm starting to feel like I can actually improve my situation. So, thanks for that!"

What I love about Donna's story is that she did lose weight but I think she gained something even more valuable. She put her head down and got to work, and her results proved to herself that she really could improve her situation. She learned to believe in herself!

The greatest obstacle to success for most people is a lack of belief in themselves. Without it, they risk suffering from...

- **A negative attitude** – We have these negative thoughts (e.g. I don't think I can do this) running around our minds, which can cripple or block our ability to focus on the positive (e.g. I can do this!).

- **Blaming others** – We don't take responsibility for our actions. We blame our genetics, our spouse, our busy schedule, and whatever else we can use as a scapegoat. When we shift responsibility, we waste precious time and energy.

- **Overwhelm** – Without belief in ourselves, we tend to get overwhelmed. And it snowballs. The more we feel overwhelmed, the worse we feel. Ultimately, it becomes a self-fulfilling prophesy and we don't get anything done. A friend of mine, Pat, is so cool, calm, and confident. Worlds could be colliding around him, but he doesn't get overwhelmed. He simply puts his energy into whatever he feels is most important. We can all learn from that.

- **Procrastination** – Once you believe in yourself you won't need to wait until New Year's to make a commitment. You'll realize the time is now!

- **Being unthankful** – When we believe in ourselves, we become more thankful. This leads to a much more rewarding and enjoyable life.

- **Apathy** – When we don't believe in ourselves, we don't bother putting energy into improving. Who cares who we surround ourselves with and where we go? We're doomed to failure anyway.

However, once people believe in themselves, their true power is unleashed and they find the resources they need to succeed. Your potential is an image of what you can become and there will be no stopping you.

Cultivate a Positive Attitude

Can attitude be cultivated? I believe it can. While some people seem to be more positive by nature, there are many techniques to being more optimistic. All of these options are tied to the same main idea:

Be thankful.

While we all have problems and things we wish were different, it's important to be grateful for what we do have. I've noticed the more grateful I become, the more I receive. I don't think that's an accident. Here are some ways to be thankful and attract more positivity into your life…

- **Say thank you** – It sounds so simple but saying thank you is a lost art. Genuinely thanking people throughout the day will make you happier. It will also brighten up the other person's day.

- **Make a list** – Here are two strategies I've used. One is to list 20 things you are thankful for. The other is to set a timer (e.g. 10 minutes) and keep writing things you're thankful for until the timer goes off. These can be done daily or as often as you'd like.

- **Pray** – If you are a person of faith, you can thank God directly. In our house, we pray before meals as well as other events (e.g. going on vacation) to thank God for what He's given us.

- **Share your list with others** – Studies show that children as young as four years old become happier if they practice gratitude early in the day. Once I learned this, I started a new tradition with my family—I had a four-year-old at the time. On the mornings we eat breakfast together, we all share three things we're thankful for. I truly believe this helps our family be more connected and positive.

Take Personal Responsibility for Your Life

One critical way to embrace a powerful mindset and set yourself up for success is to take responsibility for your life.

We all have a tendency to blame other people and our environment for our shortcomings or undesired circumstances. Whether it's the kids' activities, our negative co-workers, the economy, the president, or our parents that screwed us up, we rarely blame ourselves for our circumstances.

One of the most freeing things I've ever done was to start taking personal responsibility for my life. It's all relative, but I had problems growing up like everyone else. At a point in my early twenties, I decided to stop blaming my parents, my upbringing, my friends, or anything else for where I was at in my life. It was so liberating. I felt like I had escaped a prison—a prison in my mind. It was my choices that would determine my fate. This is when I went from being a struggling student to the top of the class. While I've certainly slipped back into the "blame game" at times, I remind myself that I can decide to try my best in any area.

Of course, past decisions by us or someone else may have consequences. That doesn't mean we can't move forward. I believe that even if we can't fully control our destiny, we should act (from an action standpoint) like we can.

In John Miller's wonderful book, *QBQ! The Question Behind the Question*, he talks about effective versus ineffective questions. We can ask ourselves certain questions to eliminate blame, victim thinking, complaining, and procrastination.

Ineffective questions begin with the words Who, Why, and When. Examples are…

- Who is responsible for this mess?

- Why can't my spouse be more supportive?

- When are things gonna go my way?

Effective (QBQ) questions begin with How or What and contain the word "I." Examples are…

- How can I help in this situation?

- What can I do to stick to my nutrition plan?

- How can I get my workout in even though I have a busy day?

Create a Positive Environment for Yourself

The environment we put ourselves in is crucial. I've been studying topics such as fitness, weight loss, and self-development for years and I don't think the concept of environment gets the attention it deserves. Your environment refers to…

- **People** – Who are you associating with? There's a saying that we are like the 5 people we spend the most time with. I think this is spot on. If you're trying to lose weight but everyone you hang around with avoids any form of exercise and eats wings and beer every day, you're headed for trouble. I'm not saying to cut off meaningful relationships. Just be mindful and intentional about who you're spending time with.

- **Food** – What kind of food is lying around at work? How about at home? You're playing with fire if you're trying to lose weight but you have a stash of cookies in the closet. Will power is overrated. Make it easier on yourself by cleaning out those cupboards.

One of our rock star clients, Will, was telling me about some pretty serious bike rides he does with the Emergency Medical Service (EMS) crew he works with. These Memorial rides honor past and present first responders. One of the 7-day rides begins in Boston and ends in Virginia.

Will's face lit up as he was telling me all about the fun, hard work, and camaraderie that goes into preparing for these events. Some of the participants have no problem with the long distances. Others do. Either way, not everyone tries to race ahead. In fact, the goal is for everyone to cross the finish line. When some of the less experienced riders are lagging, more advanced riders will "push them up," as Will says. What this means is they ride next to or behind the slower riders and encourage them to look forward and stay focused on getting ahead… a little at a time.

We all do better when we have people who care about us "pushing us up." These are the kinds of people you want to surround yourself with to set yourself up for success.

Another great example of surrounding yourself with those who lift you up comes from nature. Each year thousands of geese fly from Canada to the southern part of the US to escape the cold winter. We see them flying in V-shaped patterns with one at the front and the others in close formation. The leader actually rotates throughout their long journey. The one in charge has to expend the most energy so when it gets tired it rotates further back in the line where it can get some "lift" while another goose takes the helm.

Scientists have studied geese and their V-formation flying extensively. They've discovered that since they fly so close together in a group, they can fly 70% further than if one of them flew alone. This is due to each goose providing less wind resistance for the one behind it.

Scientists also discovered when one goose becomes sick or injured and has to drop out of formation, two other geese will drop out to take care of it.

Additionally, all the geese in the V-formation are constantly honking except one. The lead goose doesn't honk. It doesn't need to.

The other geese are honking to cheer the leader on and give encouragement. Go, goose, go!

I like to think there are similar relationships among the members of my fitness facility, Total Body Boot Camp and Performance Center (TBBC). It's not only the coaches that care; the members lift each other up as well. You'll want to find your own "flock" because no matter who you are, we all need someone behind us pushing us up and supporting us.

Face Your Challenges One Grain at a Time

Many of us feel overwhelmed and stressed about our to-do lists that never seem to end. We have families, friends, workouts, work, mortgages, bills, etc.

D. Maxwell Maltz points out in his classic book, *Psycho-Cybernetics,* that no matter how many things we have on our plate, they all come to us one at a time. We often get more overwhelmed at the thought of all we have to do rather than the items themselves. Next time this happens, think of the things you have to do as an hourglass with grains of sand falling one grain at a time. In fact, to remind myself of this principle, I bought an hourglass and put it right on my desk with a sign that reads, "One Grain at a Time."

Here is a personal example of how I had to scale things back and just focus on what was in front of me at one point.

I once had to take off from working out for 2-3 weeks. I had a nasty infection in my leg that went from bad to worse, fast. What started as a little pimple on my thigh turned into an infection that wrapped around my entire leg, putting me in the hospital on IV antibiotics. As I sat in the hospital bed for hours, it seemed like days. I wondered if and when I'd get back to my workouts.

I've never taken this long of a break. While I was tempted to go "balls to the wall" when I was cleared, I decided to be smart and ease back into things. I had to crawl before I could walk and walk before I could run, literally.

My body had to once again adapt to the physical stress after being on the couch for a few weeks. Thankfully I recovered well and was ultimately fine. By taking on the challenges as they came, one at a time, I was able to overcome them.

Be Ready for Battles You Don't Expect

Not to get too philosophical, but it seems like everyone is facing a battle. Here are some of the enemies we all might face...

- **Negative thoughts** – People need to be intentional about what they're thinking and what goes into their minds. The first step is identifying the problem. If you have self-defeating thoughts, realize that that's all they are. Just thoughts. They have no basis in reality. Hopefully this book inspires you to think and dream bigger. You can also read other books about people who achieved great success against all odds. I like to read inspirational biographies at night before bed. I try to learn about people who have made a real difference in the world. This imprints positive thoughts on my mind while I sleep. Then when I wake up I can hit the ground running trying to make a difference of my own. It really works. Just remember. There is always someone who had it much worse than you but still achieved what you set out to do. There are countless people who have lost weight and became fit and happy.

- **The media** – The media is constantly telling everyone how they should feel, how they should look, and what they should want. These are things people should decide for themselves. You are unique and have your own desires. Unfortunately, many men and women are walking around feeling insecure because they don't look like the model on the cover of the magazine. The ironic thing is that the model on the magazine cover doesn't even look like that in real life. It's all a façade. The pictures are artificially airbrushed. What's more, often times the models engage in unrealistic (dehydration) or dangerous (drugs) behavior to look a certain way for a photo shoot.

Run the race you want to run. Don't worry about anyone else. A report was given by a nurse who takes care of people when they are close to death. She asked her patients what their biggest regret was and the number one answer was: "I wish I had been true to who I was and not just lived to meet the expectations of others." You can't worry about what the media or anyone else thinks. Just be YOU and live your life without the regret of trying to be someone you're not.

- **Advertisements** – Every time I see a beer or wine commercial, there's an attractive man or woman in the ad. Rarely do they show the people that are really living that type of lifestyle (going out and drinking all the time). I wonder how the alcohol sales would be affected if the ad showed an overweight man with a bunch of teeth missing or a malnourished woman unhappy with an unfulfilled life.

  Marketing divisions of food companies are working hard competing against each other to get people's attention. Thirty billion dollars are spent every year by the food industry on advertising. What's worse, half of that is spent on advertising snack foods, candy, and soda. Unfortunately, the result is expanded waistlines.

  Advertisements vs. Kids

  Studies show that children eat 45 percent more after being exposed to snack food advertising. That's crazy! This is partly why my wife and I got rid of regular television. We'd rather help establish food preferences in our kids, not the television!

  Children are trusting and don't understand the concept of advertising. We're facing an uphill battle because the average kid sees 15 commercials about food products per day. By taking small steps, you can help protect yourself and your children from the harmful effects of advertising.

- **Friends/family** – Yes, believe it or not, the people closest to you can be the "enemy." If they're constantly making decisions that aren't in line with the life you're trying to live, that battle is very real. Sometimes they may even try to sabotage your efforts. Unfortunately, for some reason they may not want you to be thinner or healthier than they are.

  For example, I have a client. I'll call her Kim. She's a mortgage broker and co-owner of a successful business. She does private nutrition consulting with me. Kim has an excellent marriage and a beautiful family. Unfortunately, her husband Christopher doesn't have the best health habits. Christopher loves to go out to dinner and eat junk food while watching television at night. It's all in good fun, but Christopher actually jokes with Kim and tries to get her to go off of her program.

  This kind of thing can make life difficult for Kim. She wants to do the right thing, but always making the right decision can be difficult, especially when she's tired or stressed. Physical excellence takes dedication and patience. Going out to restaurants frequently and eating high fat and sugary foods regularly will sabotage results. Kim knows this so we worked out a plan.

  Kim still goes out to dinner with Christopher but only on her terms: the restaurant has some healthy options and she only goes when it fits in her plan. Kim also implemented a rule that there would be no snacking in front of the television. What's more, they now go for a 15-minute walk for every hour of TV watching. Finally, we put an accountability plan in place where Kim started sending me her nutrition plan each night. This makes a huge difference, knowing that she'll report to someone. I'm proud to say that Kim is down 6.5 pounds in just three weeks.

There can be a lot of things that are combating your efforts for a healthier life. These are just some of the ones I want you to be aware of.

Consistency Is the Key to Success

There is a common thread between the EMS bike riders, the geese, the hourglass and my layoff from workouts that I discussed in the last two sections. Slow and steady is the name of the game. As long as we are making progress each day and getting 1% better, we will reach our goals and grow. The tortoise beats the hare every time I read that story.

I like to have my clients think of weight loss like a roll of toilet paper. Think about it. If I gave you a roll of toilet paper and asked you to tear one piece off, what would happen? Would the roll look smaller? Probably not. What if I had you pull two sheets off? It still wouldn't look any different, would it? How about five? Or ten? Most likely, it still wouldn't be noticeable to the naked eye. However, if you keep pulling pieces off, eventually that roll will look smaller. In the same way, if you keep remaining consistent with your exercise and nutrition plan, eventually you will see a difference. It may just take some time.

You'll want to keep this idea of slow and steady in mind when starting and continuing your program. I will expand on the importance of consistency in Chapter 3.

CHAPTER 2:

SETTING STRONG GOALS AND REACHING THEM

WHY IS IT so important to set goals?

Everyone has different reasons for setting goals. I will share some of mine. Perhaps you will be inspired to find your own reasons.

- **Happiness** – People that set goals and achieve them are generally happier than those that don't. There is a natural high that comes with goal setting and achievement. No chemical can reproduce this feeling.

- **Reaching God-given potential** – I believe it is truly a shame not to reach our potential. Oliver Wendell Holmes Sr. said, "Most people die with their music still in them." This is really sad to me and I wouldn't want it to become a reality in my case.

- **My family and other relationships** – This is probably my biggest WHY. What I mean by my "Why" is what drives me—the deep reason for striving towards my goal. The simple things are most important to me. I am NOT driven by material things. I want to be my healthiest so I can best help the people in my life.

What are your reasons for setting goals? When you know what drives you, and especially when you are aware of your biggest WHY, you gain clarity on what makes your goals worth the challenges that come with reaching them.

There are many teachings available on goal setting. Most of them are overly complex. I've discovered a simple goal setting formula which has helped me…

- Get out of a tremendous amount of financial debt (well into six figures)

- Receive a black belt in Brazilian Jiu-jitsu

- Go back to college while working full time and graduate with honors

- Transform myself from scrawny to brawny

- Help hundreds of people achieve fitness and weight loss goals

- And much more

Setting goals is an excellent way to set yourself up for success. My formula for succeeding in reaching your goals is simple:

<u>Step One</u>: Write out your goals using the three critical guidelines for setting strong goals.

<u>Step Two</u>: Create an action plan to enable you to reach your goals.

Let me go into each one a bit more.

Step One: Use the Three Critical Guidelines to Set Strong Goals

I've always been a goal setter. In fact, here is a list of goals I made when I was 12 years old.

1. Try earring (I thought it was cool)

2. Eat like mad (I wanted to gain weight)

3. Get closer to God (I wanted to do the right thing)

I didn't say I was always good at goal setting. It's funny to look at that list now. While I was much better off setting the goals above than not doing so, there are three main ways I failed to make my goals as strong as possible. In order to make your goals the strongest statements of intention you can, you want to use these *three critical guidelines*…

1. **Make your goals specific** – Goals should be specific because they will have a much greater chance of success than a general goal. An example of a general goal is, "Get in shape." A specific goal would be "Lose 15 pounds." You'll want to set specific goals so you know when you've accomplished them. If you set a general goal of "Lose weight," what happens if you lose an ounce? You might not be satisfied even though you technically "lost weight." My second goal, "Eat like mad," is not specific. A better one might have been, "Eat 5 meals per day consisting of high quality protein and complex carbs."

2. **Make your goals measurable** – All goals should have a date attached to them. A goal without a deadline is just a dream. In my above example, I could have said, "Get an earring before July 1." Having a target date to reach your goal will create some healthy pressure to keep you on track. It's OK if you don't hit your goal in time. You'll still be further along than if you hadn't set the goal in the first place.

3. **State your goals in the present tense** – Goals should be stated in the present tense. This way you can visualize it as a reality. Growing up in a Christian home, I wanted to have a better relationship with God. A present tense version of number 3 might be, "My goal is to pray every day." Or, to make it even more specific: "My goal is to pray every night before bed."

By incorporating these three guidelines into your goal setting, your likelihood to succeed in reaching your goals increases dramatically.

An additional guideline that I recommend when setting goals is to include the word "I." This makes the statement even more active. "I will pray every day." "I will get an earring before July 1." "I will eat five meals per day consisting of…." This simple act of making your goal into an "I" statement causes you to take further ownership of the goal.

To go even further, I recommend that you *turn your goals into affirmations.*

Many people find that they do even better by acting "as if" they have already reached their goal. They do this by turning their goals into a statement that makes the goal real to them. Reflecting two of my above examples, you might write "I pray every evening" or "I eat five meals per day."

As another example, instead of saying "Lose 15 pounds," you might say "I am a healthy and fit 120 (or whatever the ideal weight is) pounds" or "I am in the process of becoming a healthy and fit 120 pounds."

The idea behind making your goal into an affirmation is that we will act according to what we think is reality. If you see yourself as a healthy and fit 120-pounder, you'll want to make decisions in line with that goal.

Words are powerful, so if you say things like "I want to lose 15 pounds" you may just become more aware of the fact that you're heavier than you want to be. This may cause you to focus more on the fact that you're 15 pounds overweight than on your objective of becoming the healthy weight you want to be.

Creating an affirmation from a goal is simple. Put the word "I" in it and place it in the present tense. For example, if your goal is to eat a healthy breakfast, an affirmation might be, "I eat a healthy breakfast each day."

Now that you know how to set strong goals, let's move on to Step 2.

Step Two: Create an Action Plan to Reach Your Goals

Once you have clearly written, strong, specific goals, you'll need an action plan that will enable you to reach them.

To create an action plan, write out the specific action steps you plan to take that will allow you to reach your goal. These action steps need to be clear and measurable, and they need to lead directly to your goal.

You want to keep these steps simple. Don't get caught up in a grand analysis of every single step imaginable needed to reach your goal. Start small with 1-3 main steps that reaching your goal will require.

Examples of Strong Goals and Action Plans

Below I outline a few fitness related examples of making a strong goal and action plan. In the examples I also add a target date. The target date would depend on how far you are currently from the goal. In my examples, I think 30 days would be reasonable for most people.

Example #1

Goal: I will perform a perfect push-up within 30 days. (Or as an affirmation: I am performing the perfect push-up.)

Action Plan:

1. I will learn the proper technique from my coach.

2. I will practice the proper technique three times per week.

3. I will do planks on "off" days to strengthen my core.

Target Date: January 5 (or 30 days from the start date)

Example #2

Goal: I will lose five pounds. (Or as an affirmation: I am in the process of becoming a healthy and fit 155 pounds.)

Action Plan:

1. I will eat breakfast daily.

2. I will keep a food journal.

3. I will plan my meals in advance.

Target Date: January 5 (or 30 days from the start date)

Example #3

Goal: I will get to the gym three times per week. (Or as an affirmation: I go to the gym three times a week.)

Action Plan:

1. I will schedule my sessions in my appointment calendar.

2. I will get my workout clothes ready the night before.

3. I will meet a buddy at the gym.

Target Date: January 5 (or 30 days from the start date)

Setting Smart Goals Beyond Fitness

While the focus of this book is fitness and weight loss, we should also have goals in the following areas.

- Financial (e.g. I save $50 each month for my travel fund)

- Spiritual (e.g. I pray each morning for 10 minutes)

- Relationships/Social (e.g. My spouse and I discuss what is on our hearts every Sunday evening)

- Intellectual (e.g. I read a book a month)

- Career (e.g. I set 5 sales appointments each week)

- Family (e.g. I have dinner with my family at least 5 days a week)

Don't forget to include a target date and an action plan, as demonstrated in the fitness goal examples in the above section. If you haven't done so yet, let's do it now. Like right now. Before you move on. I'll wait. List the following…

- Goal (be specific)

- Category (e.g. fitness)

- Action steps needed to complete goal

- Target date

Keep Your Vision in Front of You

Studies tell us that we move closer to what we consistently look at. It's important to have something in front of you, even if it's purely symbolic, to remind you of what you're striving for.

A struggling actor who once lived in his car wrote a check to himself for 10 million dollars for "acting services rendered," post-dated it for 10 years, and tucked it in his wallet. What was unusual about this was that he wrote this check during a period when he was struggling to get parts.

During tough times he would sit up on the hills of Hollywood and look at the check. About 12 years later he starred in *Dumb and Dumber* and *Batman Forever* and earned a combined 14 million dollars! Yes, I'm talking about Jim Carey.

Do you have your version of a 10 million dollar check?

It's so helpful to keep your goals, visions, and dreams in front of you. Put pictures around your house to remind yourself. Are there sayings or quotes that inspire you? Put those up as well! You'll be amazed how these constant reminders can help keep you focused.

One of the areas my wife Melissa and I struggled with in the past was our finances. As we worked through our mountain of debt, there were many ups and downs. While we made great progress some months, there were others we didn't have any extra to throw at the credit card, medical, or student-loan debt. The biggest loan we paid off was a whopping $64,000. We knew we needed something visual to keep us focused. We decided to make a chart that we would fill in each time we made a payment. We eventually put other pictures around the house to remind us of our dreams.

It's important to have a visual reminder in front of you regardless of what you're working towards. The same strategy that helped us with our finances can help you with fitness or weight loss.

One of our members at Total Body Boot Camp and Performance Center, Kristen, started out with a goal to lose 15 pounds and be consistent with her fitness routine. She had tried other solutions. She just never stuck with anything long enough to reap the rewards. Things were different at TBBC. The sense of community and fun kept her coming back.

Kristen, a nurse in her forties, is in the best shape of her life now. Not only is she down 15 pounds but her endurance has improved so much that she can now run 3 miles and do 50 push-ups.

One of the things that helped keep her inspired was changing the screen saver on her phone to a picture of a fitness model. Every time she feels like giving up, she looks at her phone and is motivated to keep working. This especially helps her at work. Her phone is always nearby, so when she's tempted to eat something less than optimal, she sees the picture on her phone and skips the junk food!

It's so easy to get caught up in the day to day and lose sight of the bigger picture. You'll want to take some specific actions to keep your vision in front of you and remember what you're working towards.

CHAPTER 3:

MOTIVATION AND ABOVE ALL, CONSISTENCY

THERE'S A LOT of talk on motivation nowadays. Motivation is great but it often fades. In this chapter, we'll take a look at how to motivate yourself but even more importantly, how to remain consistent. As discussed in brief in Chapter 1, consistency is the key to your success. With the right actions performed consistently over time, there will be no stopping you.

"People often say that motivation doesn't last. Well, neither does bathing—that's why we recommend it daily."
– Zig Ziglar

The hard part with weight loss or any behavioral change is not so much the initial part of the process—that's kind of fun and exciting. It's when life knocks you down and you have to get up and keep going that presents the greater challenge. While many people begin a fitness or weight loss program because of a short-term goal like a wedding or vacation, there needs to be a long-term plan. This way you don't wind up like two-thirds of people who lose weight—right back to where you were a couple of years (or less) later.

It's the strangest thing when people work hard to get the results they were seeking and then quit. I first noticed this phenomenon early in my career. Now that I've been helping people transform their bodies and lives for almost 20 years, I know it happens all the time.

A guy named Arthur signed on with me and was laser focused. He wanted to lose his love handles and feel better about himself. He also thought it would help his career. Arthur really seemed to have his head in the right place from what I could tell. His goals were well defined, he had a solid reason why he wanted to achieve them, and he seemed ready to work.

He followed my program to a tee. Arthur was a man on a mission. Conditioning every day? No problem. He was in the gym on a regular basis getting his butt kicked and loving it. Sugar-free diet? Done. He was definitely willing to sacrifice in order to succeed.

As time went on, you're probably wondering if Arthur changed. Did his love handles disappear? Did his confidence improve? Did he get a promotion at work? Well, let me tell you. The answer to all three questions is yes. He put forth the effort and got the results. In just 12 short weeks, his love handles were no longer noticeable. He was coming in regularly with a huge smile on his face and feeling great.

Everything seemed to be fine and dandy, but let me tell you what happened next. Arthur started to slip back into his old habits. His healthy oatmeal breakfast was replaced with pop tarts and other high sugar foods. What's more, he no longer seemed enthused about his workouts or his goals.

Unfortunately, he not only put back on the weight and then some but his love handles became bigger than ever. His self-confidence dipped to an all-time low and he ended up with even more health problems. Ugh. So frustrating and disappointing. I saw him busting his butt each day. His hard work was paying off and my heart broke as I witnessed his decline. It almost brings tears to my eyes now as I think about how success slipped through his fingers.

Let's look at what actually happened. Based on what I see all too often, there are several possibilities why Arthur didn't stay motivated or consistent. As crazy as it seems, some people are scared of success. It takes them out of their comfort zone. Perhaps Arthur was comfortable being soft and the prospect of a new physique was just too much to handle. Or perhaps he had trouble seeing himself as he was now, healthy and fit. Even though he had transformed his body, he still thought of himself as unfit and unhealthy. Eventually his actions followed his thoughts.

Additionally, Arthur may have had some false expectations of how these changes would impact his life. I know he was disappointed that his transformation didn't inspire his wife to lose weight.

We also know that habits are delicate. Arthur had some very unhealthy influences in his life and eventually they drew him back. As the saying goes, "Old habits die hard." The bottom line is, Arthur failed to realize that…

Behavioral change is NOT permanent.

That's the big takeaway. It's like saying a wealthy person doesn't have to be responsible with money. Nothing can be further from the truth. The wealthy person must continue to be responsible with money. That's how they became wealthy in the first place. If they want to stay wealthy, the habits must remain. This is why most lotto winners can win millions and revert back to the same level of wealth (and happiness) in just two short years.

We must follow up on our new changes. If not, our positive results won't last. Once we hit our fitness goals, we must be intentional about maintaining them. The commitment and discipline need to remain.

I hope you're prepared to go to the gym—forever.

Motivation and "Why" Power

Ask yourself why you want to be healthy and fit. Sure, we all want to look better, but perhaps there is a deeper reason? I'm going to refer to this deeper reason as your "why." It's worth taking the time to discover your **why**. Without a strong why we tend to give up when the going gets tough. What's going to keep you from grabbing that bag of chips after a long day at work? Your **why** can if it's strong enough. My why is my family. I have other powerful reasons too. I love the way I feel when I'm fit and healthy. I love to do jiu-jitsu and need to be healthy to do so. I want to be a good example for our Warriors (that's what we call our clients). All of those reasons are great but nothing trumps my quest to be there (in optimal shape) for my family. This is what will help me get up at 4 a.m. to make sure I have time for a workout.

Here are some examples of **whys** I've seen from some of my more successful clients.

- **To be there for their kids** – Parents want to be healthy so they can be around for their kids. They also want to set a good example for their children.

- **To truly live life** – As sad as it is, many people are just going through the motions. To truly live life how it's meant to be lived, you'll want to be fit and healthy. This way you can be fully engaged with life and all its ups and downs. You'll not only be in the game but you'll be winning.

- **To avoid pain** – We are either running towards pleasure or away from pain. Perhaps a medical scare is motivating you to get healthier and/or lose weight. Many of our clients have completely transformed themselves as a result of a medical scare.

I wonder how Arthur would have made out had he had a deeper why such as these. Looking better is great, but the deeper we can connect our reason to our goal, the higher our chance of success will be.

Medical Motivation: A New Lease on Life

I was once diagnosed with diabetes. It turned out to be a huge mistake (my lab report got mixed up with someone else's), which is a different story for a different day. For one full week I believed that I had diabetes and that my life would be forever changed by this bully of a disease. Since I knew how badly I wanted to be around for my family, I immediately (after a dose of denial and grief) began eating as close to a perfect diet as possible. I jotted every meal down and refused to miss an effective meal free from sugar. The interesting thing was that it wasn't hard. My "why" or deep core reason for pursuing health was so strong that even a little bit of sugar wasn't worth it.

We are all motivated by different things. As mentioned above, it's important to spend some time discovering yours. One client of mine named Rosanne told me what motivated her. She needed minor surgery. The doctor's office called to let her know that she would need to have the surgery at the hospital rather than the doctor's office. The reason was because she was considered a higher risk because her Body Mass Index (BMI) was so high. Your BMI is used to determine obesity. This was the catalyst for Roseanne to start training with us and join our nutrition program.

Medical scares can not only motivate people to change their health behaviors in a positive way but make the changes stick for the long-term.

The Power of a Strong "Why": Sonji

Sonji had never made New Year's Resolutions before because she knew they rarely worked. She waited until mid-January to ensure she was serious. After reflecting on how out of shape she'd gotten, she decided to do something about it. She had transformed herself once years ago but was ready to make it stick this time. She needed a place of encouragement, motivation, and inspiration. She said she knew she found the right place when she received a call back from one of our Directors of First Impressions, Sam. Sonji described Sam's energy as infectious.

Sonji had recently turned 50 and was fed up over how she had let herself go. She would get winded after walking up a flight of stairs. She came to us weighing 207 pounds and could not run across the floor without becoming extremely fatigued. It was a slow go for her because she couldn't handle much physically at first. She simply took one step at a time and kept at it. Three months later, it was quite a celebration when she was able to do 10 sprints back and forth across the floor. She improved her endurance by doing just a little more than her body was used to each week. Sonji now weighs a healthy 140 pounds and is feeling great. She can do things now that she couldn't have imagined, such as sprinting, squatting with weights, push-ups, and burpees. She even fit back into clothes she kept in her closet for 3 years! As Sonji put it, "TBBC has helped me to rediscover the inner being at my core by helping me realize that in order to take care of anyone else, I must first take care of myself."

Sonji had the mental clarity and dedication to keep herself motivated. She finally learned to take care of herself first. Knowing she had to prioritize her health in order to take care of those she loved kept her fire burning to reach her goals and beyond.

Motivated by Others: Clarice

Another member named Clarice came in and had similar goals as Sonji. Clarice had tried a bunch of times over the years to lose weight. Unfortunately she always attempted to lose weight with programs she couldn't maintain. I taught Clarice to surround herself with people doing what she wants (i.e. becoming fit and healthy). Clarice immediately connected with Sonji. She was inspired by Sonji's story and they even worked out together. In fact, check out what Clarice had to say about the experience.

> "When I met Sonji in group training over a year ago, I could immediately tell that she was a kind and good-hearted person. When Billy would run us over to the park for a training, Sonji and I were the slowest, so we kept each other company, and we'd chat as we jogged our way there and back. In addition to being kind, she had a very calm determination about her, and she was clear about what she wanted for herself regarding her health and fitness. About a year ago, Sonji and I sat next to each other during the first meeting for the Spring Answers (a nutrition accountability group) program. During the Answers program I would look forward (and still do!) to her motivational Facebook posts and words of encouragement.

"Fast-forward to earlier this year: I had to go on medical leave from Total Body Boot Camp and hadn't seen Sonji in months. The first time I saw her again, it was literally a do-a-double-take, jaw-falling-to-the-floor moment. She had achieved her fitness goals and looked amazing...like the best version of herself. I realized that she and I had started out at the same time and place, were about the same age, and had probably been about the same fitness level, but Sonji had kept her eye on her why, and she had done what I dream of doing. That calm determination had kept her doing what she needed to do to get what she wanted.

"It's not that I've never seen anyone transform themselves before, but I guess it was that Sonji and I had started out at the same starting line, but she had kept running the race. When the notification for the nutrition accountability group came that spring, I thought back to a year ago, and thought, 'If I had done what Sonji did, I would be where she is, and if I now do what she did, next year I too can be where she is, and where I want to be.' She didn't stop when Answers ended; she kept going, knowing that slow and steady wins the race. She had an unshakeable faith that she was going to succeed at her goal, and she did. And not only that, her support and example have now given me the faith to do it, too."

Clarice realized that if Sonji could do it, so could she. Sonji told Clarice it was never too late to achieve what she wanted. Now Clarice is on her way! As of this writing, she's down 10 pounds.

Health scares like Rosanne had can be one way a person is motivated. Some, like Sonji, are motivated by their "why" power—in her case knowing that she had to take care of herself first in order to best take care of those in her care. Some, like Clarice, are inspired by other people. We are all uniquely motivated but discovering that reason is crucial, like finding a key to a unique lock.

Consistency in Eating Healthy

Consistently eating healthy is critical, whether your goal is to lose weight, to gain muscle, to improve your health, or to perform better. Often it feels difficult to choose the healthier option day in and day out. Food boredom kicks in, and with it so does your sweet tooth. It can be a challenge to figure out how to consistently make choices that bring you closer to your goals. Most of us have spent most of our lives making food choices that are less than ideal. Changing our mental programming of the last twenty, thirty, or forty-plus years requires diligence and mindfulness, day in and day out. We are literally forging a new pathway in our brain to learn to eat eggs and vegetables in the morning versus the Pop Tarts of our youth. We will inevitably slip up, and that is okay. The key is consistency, not perfection.

Speaking of consistency, you'll hear different statistics about how much of weight loss is due to exercise versus how much is due to nutrition. Some experts say 80/20 and some say 75/25 both in favor of nutrition. Yes, you can lose weight with just adding exercise but your results will be dramatically improved by eating the right amounts of the right foods. We often tell our members, "You can't out-exercise a bad diet."

When it comes to eating consistently, what I have learned is…

What Gets Written Gets Done

Studies show that one of the most common habits among people that get fit and stay that way is writing down what they eat. Here are some ideas to make this work for you.

- **Plan ahead** – Don't get caught hungry. Plan ahead so you know you'll have a better option available. Plan your meals the night before. Have healthy, last-resort snacks available in your car, in your desk at work, or in your pantry.

- **Jot it down before you eat it** – One of the worst ways to journal is by trying to remember what you had that day and then writing it down. Writing it down beforehand will truly help improve your behavior. There are apps (e.g. MyFitness-Pal) that allow you to track this digitally.

- **Report yourself** – Get some accountability. Share your journal with someone you trust. Or share it with a qualified coach.

Next Level Tracking

Once you get the basics down you can begin implementing the following check mark system that has worked wonders for our coaching clients. We call it Next Level Tracking.

Once you finish your tracking for the day, take the following steps.

1. Reflect for a minute or two on what you did well and what you could have improved.

2. Give yourself a check mark for each effective meal (i.e. lean protein, fibrous veggie w/ or w/o starchy carb)

3. Give yourself a dash for each meal that was less than effective (e.g. the meal contained simple sugar)

4. Give yourself an X for any meals that you missed.

5. Calculate your percentage of check marks.

The goal is to have 90% check marks. Most of us have a lot of work to do. This is OK. We are looking for gradual improvements. The magic is in doing just a bit better each day.

Remember you get what you put in. The more you track the better you'll do. It's actually pretty simple, but so few people do the simple things it takes to improve. You're different though, right?

Success boils down to a few behaviors done properly and consistently day in and day out.

Remember to never give up. Ever.

Action Steps

Action breeds success. In Chapter 2 I discussed making a list of action steps for each of your goals, so you have a plan for success. If your goal is to eat healthier, here are three simple action steps you can start doing that will have a major IMPACT in the near and long term.

1. Journal each meal before consuming it.

2. Report it to a friend or coach.

3. Learn from it and grow.

*If the terminology for an effective meal is confusing, we'll clear that up in *Chapter 9: A Simple Plan for Making Healthy Food Choices.*

**If the above system for tracking seems a bit too complex, don't fret. I will share an even simpler method for giving yourself the accountability you need on a daily basis. Look out for it in the next chapter: *Choosing Success Over Self-Sabotage.*

As with most things, the key to greater success lies in planning. Of course there is the doing, which we will address, but we need a solid plan. Change is hard and a solid plan will give you the confidence and tools you need to win!

When life is going smoothly and there aren't any major problems, things tend to work out. It's scenarios like this that can derail us...

- An argument with a loved one

- A "crisis" at work

- We miss a few days because of a life event and lose our momentum.

Studies show that when people prepare ahead of time with a written plan for how they will handle a potential problem, they are much more likely to succeed.

This is something that has to be specific to your potential obstacle.

You might write something like this:

"When I'm at the party I'll sit far away from the dessert table. I will not stand around the food area to talk to people. I will have no more than one normal serving size. I will remember my goal, how important it is to me, and how hard I've worked. I will not sabotage this."

This doesn't mean you have to be perfect or can never have any dessert. It just means that you have a plan. You will do far better this way than if you didn't have a written plan.

Consistency in Working Out

As I said before: I hope you're prepared to go to the gym—forever.

If you want to get results and maintain them, if you want to cultivate a strong and fit body, if you want to maximize your health and life on this earth—stay active.

The best way to stay active is to find something you love. Even better is if you do it with a group that will keep you accountable. Check out a boot camp near you. Look into different activities and gyms that appeal to you. Try new things. You might be surprised at what you discover you love. Check out Brazilian Jiu-Jitsu, kickboxing, cycling, pilates, yoga, indoor rock climbing, or tennis. Find a running or hiking group near you. If you're in a rural area, look into online training groups. If you have very limited time, look into 10-minute or 20-minute workout videos on YouTube or elsewhere online.

Strive to do some sort of activity every, or on most days. Incorporate variety to keep things fresh and exciting. Here is what a sample week might look like. This may or may not be realistic for you. Don't get too caught up in that right now. Just use it as a model.

Monday –   Group class at a local gym
Tuesday –   Strength training
Wednesday – Something restorative like stretching or yoga
Thursday -   Group class at a local gym
Friday –   Strength training
Saturday –   Something restorative like stretching or yoga
Sunday –   Long walk, light jog, or some fun family activity
                      (e.g. soccer at a local park)

There are many, many options. You're sure to have fun with something.

Of course, sometimes it doesn't feel as fun. That's okay, too. You don't always have to love getting up at 5:30 a.m. to go do burpees and push-ups. That's when you keep your "Why" in mind and do it anyway.

Harnessing the Power of Momentum

You ever notice how certain people tend to get better and better? Certain things just seem to go their way. Part of this is due to momentum.

Just imagine someone pushing a big boulder up a hill. She gives it a push and not much happens. A little more pushing though and she finally gets the thing rolling. At this point, the person has to give maximum effort to get that momentum going. Once it's going she continues to push but it becomes much easier. If she keeps pushing with the same intensity, it really builds up speed and goes faster and faster.

You can develop the same momentum with your new routine. You just have to start pushing. Once you do, you'll be unstoppable. You can't stop pushing, though. To develop and maintain your routine you'll have to do it regularly, ideally every day.

Perseverance

You have to really want to succeed in order to persevere. You must determine that you will keep going no matter what.

Meet Tina. Tina is one of our Warriors in her mid-thirties who knows about perseverance. She had been training with us for over a year and was frustrated because the pounds didn't come off like she'd hoped. Like a lot of people she measured her progress using the scale. Each morning she would wake up and step on her scale. When that needle didn't move, she felt defeated. And she lost very little weight in the first few months. This was hard to deal with because she always put so much stock into the number on the scale. Even though she was discouraged, she kept a positive attitude and never stopped believing.

In that year she also had some personal setbacks, including the loss of a job as well as a bad break up. We all know how stressful both of these events can be. Struggling in three of life's most important areas—career, health, and relationships—was not easy and each day was a battle for her.

She wanted to quit but my team and I encouraged her to keep going. We spent some extra time talking to her at the facility. We called her and wrote messages. We wanted her to know we believed in her. Tina went on to lose 25 pounds following our program. She also is in a new and better relationship and has a fantastic job. She's happier than ever. Tina is proof that we can overcome the trials in our life and come out stronger.

All successful people experience some adversity. Actually, all people experience adversity. It's the successful ones that overcome it and get better as a result. Don't make the mistake of thinking it'll be easy. Just know that all you overcome will make it that much sweeter.

Practical Tips for Staying Motivated and Consistent

I'll end this chapter with some practical tips you can resort to when the going gets tough.

- **Stay inspired** – Read about other people who accomplished what you're setting out to. If you can't find any, let me know. We have dozens of showcases I can share – like Frank, who lost 100 pounds in one short year!

- **Cut things out** – Perhaps you're having a hard time staying focused because you're doing too much. Limit your activities to the essential to make sure you're focusing on what's truly important.

- **Do something** – Many times we get overwhelmed and end up doing nothing. For example, since we don't have the 45 minutes we need to work out, we skip it altogether. We completely ignore the fact that something is better than nothing.

- **Pump yourself up** – Memorize some mantras you can use. Think about the ideal version of yourself who has completed the goal. Get excited. It may sound corny but it works.

- **Phone a friend** – Get some support for added accountability. Tell them your pain point or what you're struggling with. Even better, get a qualified coach.

- **Stay positive** – Don't accept what Zig Ziglar called "stinkin thinkin." Squash those thoughts that don't serve you and replace them with positive ones.

- **Give yourself grace** – You won't be perfect. You won't always feel super motivated. That's OK. Just keep going.

I know you can do this. If you've read this far into the book, you're serious about your goals and I congratulate you. Keep going. I believe in you!

Bonus Tip – Studies show that people who have the built-in accountability of working out with others are 37% more likely to succeed. It's this very reason that we're so intentional about building a strong sense of community at our facilities. People come and everyone knows their name--like *Cheers*. People care. If they don't show up, they'll get a phone call.

For instance, I received this message from Kim on our Facebook page:

> *After close to a 4 week hiatus, riddled with "good" excuses, I made it back to TBBC today. I want to thank Samantha Gilchrist for the "where have you been" voice mail, Billy Hofacker for his post on those who lose their way (I didn't want to be one of them), and Billy Powers for the awesome workout this morning - All reasons why I love this place. Their commitment to their clients is second to none!!! Thank you to all.*

We all need support and guidance. It's foolish to think we can do it on our own. I'm so honored to be a part of Kim's journey. By the way, she lost 15 pounds in 6 weeks.

CHAPTER 4:

CHOOSING SUCCESS OVER SELF-SABOTAGE

IN THIS CHAPTER I'll discuss some areas you can control to create your own destiny. We will explore how to make the right decisions as well as how to set up your surroundings for success.

Don't say, "If I could I would." Say instead, "If I can, I will."
— Jim Rohn

Lynne came to me frustrated. She explained that she had lost 10 pounds on one program, 15 on another, 7 working with a trainer, and 12 on Weight Watchers. As she was explaining all the weight she had lost to me, I was trying to add it up in my head. I was up to over 40 pounds but was confused. Lynne only had about 10 pounds to lose. 20 at most. Then I realized what was going on. She had lost weight on all of the different programs but had gained it all back. It's the typical yo-yo cycle. You go on one program and it works in the short term but then the weight comes back and then some. This usually happens with calorie deprivation type programs. These are plans where you eat very little. Lynne didn't realize it but over time her metabolism was slowing and she became prone to storing more body fat.

Lynne has stuck with us for a year, which is longer than she's stuck with any other fitness program. She followed the strategies we laid out for her and finally achieved her goal of being in great shape. I am so proud of her. In this chapter, I'll explain some of the strategies we've used with Lynne and others to prevent them from sabotaging their own fitness goals.

As you'll see, much of what we address with weight loss comes down to mindset. That's why so much of the first few chapters is dedicated to this topic.

We Will Never Out-Perform Our Self-Image

When I first started out coaching people with their fitness, I noticed some folks would do phenomenally well while others seemed to struggle. I knew that if I could figure out the key difference between the two I would be able to help more people and find more fulfillment in my career. This is when I started exploring other resources outside of the fitness industry. I read books from men like Zig Ziglar and John Maxwell. Doing this, I learned a concept that changed my life. I had an "Aha moment." Reading something in a book is one thing, but seeing it play out in your life is a different story. I am absolutely certain that this concept is one of the biggest reasons for success or failure.

Concept: *We will never out-perform our self-image.*

In other words, if you see yourself as "fat," you'll do what fat people do. In order to succeed, you need to start seeing yourself as the ideal version of you. In other words, paint the picture of how you want to look and feel in your mind. Use your imagination. How do you look? What are you wearing? How do others see you? What is your energy like? Once you have this picture in your mind, you can use it to keep yourself focused. It's almost like it's guaranteed and now it's just a matter of time.

A lot of the decisions we make are a result of how we see ourselves. If we see ourselves as fat or not good enough we'll purchase cookies and chips at the supermarket. After all, to our mind, that's what those kinds of people do. However, if we see ourselves as fit and healthy, we'll make different choices. We'll do what healthy, fit, and confident people do. We'll go to the gym and make healthy food choices. The key is to change how we see ourselves.

Think about that for a minute. It's powerful. How do you see yourself?

There are two main examples in my own life that come to mind when I think of this concept that we will never out-perform our self-image. The first involves getting out of debt, and the second involves my academic success in college.

Example #1: Getting Out of Debt

I mentioned in the last chapter that one of the things I accomplished through goal setting was becoming debt free (other than my house). This was no small feat. My wife and I had accumulated tens of thousands of dollars in debt. I'm talking well into the six figures. Credit cards. Medical bills. Student loans. You name it.

We were close to throwing in the towel because we felt so defeated. This is when we got really mad. We were fed up. We decided to do something about it.

There are two points to this story. One is us hitting rock bottom. That was the sound of the tow truck hauling away my white Honda Accord that Monday morning. I didn't know how I'd get to work. My car had been repossessed. Like a lot of other people, I had to have something like this happen to get mad enough to change. It was a wake-up call.

The second thing I want to point out is our mindset. We saw ourselves as broke because we were. I can assure you we were not in denial. At the same time, this is why we stayed broke for so long. Our perspective of ourselves as being stuck in debt perpetuated our continuing to be stuck in debt. We never saw ourselves as poor though. Being "poor" is more of a spirit. A spirit of self-defeat—a that's-just-the-way-it-is type of thing.

The beginning of changing our situation was to change our perspective. We said enough was enough and we chose to see ourselves as capable and committed, and we imagined ourselves as debt free. I truly believe this difference in our mindset is what helped enable us to put one foot in front of the other and claw ourselves free from the bondage of debt.

Trust me when I say my wife and I are no different from you. We had a modest income. What we had in our favor was contentment and a lack of a need to try and keep up with the Joneses. In five short years we were able to go from being completely broke and almost on the street to being debt free besides our mortgage. We have a six-month emergency fund, college plans for our girls, a healthy retirement account, enough to give, and even some left over for fun.

If we could accomplish this big scary goal with our finances, you can take on whatever health, fitness, or weight loss challenge you're facing, no matter how overwhelming it may seem!

Example #2: Seeing Myself as an Academic Success

In high school, I was a mediocre student at best. My grades were decent before high school but even then I never saw school as "my thing." I was more interested in goofing off and excelling in sports. I was serious about those things.

I did what I needed to get by but that was it. I even switched out of the more challenging classes to be with my friends at one point. I remember reading about scholar athletes and being so impressed. "Wow, they are both superstar athletes and academic successes," I thought. "How talented they are. How do they do it? I wish I could do that." I never once thought or believed I could.

Fast forward a few years to community college. I met someone who would become a good friend: Justin. Here was someone I thought was cool. He was different than the other "cool" kids I knew, though. He actually cared about his grades and his future. In fact, after one of our anatomy tests, he went up to the professor to ask for clarification on a question he had gotten wrong. When he got back to his seat I noticed his score. A 98! I was happy with my 72 and never thought to ask the professor for any help.

The more I got to know Justin, the more I realized how similar we actually were. We both loved basketball. We had a similar sense of humor. We really clicked. His positive qualities started rubbing off on me. There was one difference between us, though. Up to this point in our lives, he had experienced much more adversity. He had come from an abusive home and both of his parents were deaf. I couldn't imagine.

Although I had my own struggles, I still lived at home and my mom made my lunch each day. Justin lived on his own, in Harlem. He had a 2-hour-plus commute to school, which meant he had to get up before 4 a.m. to start his day. He didn't get home until late in the evenings.

Something started to click with me. Justin encouraged me. He said, "Billy, you could do as well as I do if not better. You just have to put the effort in."

Sometimes you need a lift from someone else to see your own capacity. Justin's encouragement helped me realize that I could indeed excel academically, although before him the possibility had never occurred to me.

Around this time, I also received life-changing encouragement from my college math professor, Dr. Skurnick. Dr. Skurnick was different than any teacher I'd had. He was so patient and kind. He made complicated material simple to grasp. He actually managed to make college math fun. He would do silly things like try to rap. One day I was at his office for extra help since I was struggling to catch up with my academics. This was the price I had to pay due to goofing off in high school. I was trying to change my ways when I received a compliment that changed the entire course of my life. In the middle of Dr. Skurnick helping me with a problem, he paused, looked up at me and said, "Billy, you know I have these office hours to help students twice per week and you're the only one that ever comes. You seem like the type of guy that can do anything you put your mind to."

Wow! I couldn't believe it. He was talking about me. This was a very smart man, a Ph. D. in mathematics.

With Justin and Dr. Skurnick's encouragement, I was able to look at myself in an entirely new light. Before, it never occurred to me that I could be an academic success, so academic success eluded me. *I could not out-perform my self-image.* After they got through to me, I was able to perceive myself as academically capable, so I was able to become academically successful. From there, everything shifted.

I began modeling Justin's study habits and schedule. I gained confidence and started believing in myself. It wasn't easy. I had a lot of work to do. I spent countless hours studying and going for extra help. Over time, I became the student that the others went to for help. Ultimately I graduated from college, Cum Laude. I wondered if my former high school peers and teachers would even recognize me!

Sometimes You Just Need a Lift

Sometimes we just need someone to speak truth and encouragement into our lives. That's what Justin and Dr. Skurnick did for me. I'd like to do the same for you so here goes...

YOU have what it takes to become the person you want to be. I believe in you. Now get to it!

Changing Our Perspective

Remember, when we change the way we look at things, the things we look at change.

Take a look at this picture.

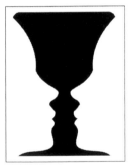

What do you see?

Is it two faces? Or is it a vase? Or do you see both? How long did it take you to see them?

When some people see this picture they see two faces right away. Others see a vase or a chalice.

It takes some people longer to see.

The point is we all see things differently. Who is right?

How about this picture?

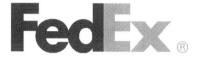

Let me know when you see the arrow. I'll wait. Some people see it right away. Others take a bit longer. It took me a while when I was first shown it, but now I'll never look at a FedEx logo the same.

Hint: The arrow is between the E and the X.

Henry Ford once said, "Whether you think you can, or you think you can't—you're right."

Again, when we change the way we look at things, the things we look at change.

This is one of the biggest "secrets" known to man.

All of our actions originate with thoughts. We eventually do things subconsciously because of beliefs or paradigms we have. A paradigm is a perspective for how we see something.

Most people get this all wrong and don't realize how important their thoughts are. They just let their thoughts control them and sort of go with the flow.

Thoughts matter. If we are going to have success in any area we need to learn to check them.

I attended a Dr. Gary Smalley seminar once and he said that thoughts are trees. Positive thoughts are big branches with lots of leaves that grow lots of fruit. Negative thoughts are little unhealthy twigs.

Every thought matters and each one begets another. Similar thoughts grow similar branches and so the pattern goes. Are you growing healthy branches with plenty of fruit or little twigs?

How Can We Change Our Thoughts?

This all sounds good, but how can we change our thoughts? Here are a few ways that have worked for me and the people I've worked with.

First things first. *Change your environment.* Charlie "Tremendous" Jones said, "You are the same as you'll be in five years except for two things; the books you'll read and the people you'll meet." Are the people you spend time with growing you or setting you back? How do you feel when you're with them?

Next, *see the possibilities.* Start with a small accomplishment and think about what good will happen when small victories start adding up. Remember, Rome wasn't built in a day and neither will the new you!

Finally, *practice gratitude.* Share three things you're thankful for each day or list them in a notebook and see how much your attitude and life can change.

Even reading this you may be having certain thoughts. Think about two possible thought scenarios. Which do you think would produce better results?

Here's your first choice in the way you can think. "I'm going to do this! I know there are things I take for granted, so starting today I'll be intentional about recognizing them. I also know that if I have a plan and start taking small steps, good things will happen. I'm going to surround myself with encouraging people that lift me up and I will pour into them in return."

Or, you can think, "Yeah, yeah. I saw this on Oprah once and it didn't work. What's the point anyway? Nothing ever goes my way."

It's obvious which scenario is better, but it's not necessarily easy to take inventory of your thoughts. Just remember, thoughts become things! Be mindful of them.

I recently read a book about George H.W. Bush written by his son, George W. Bush, called *41.* Regardless of what you think regarding the political career of the former Bush, there is no doubt that he had a very colorful life. If you're like me, you tend to think that some people just get all the breaks. We look at someone like George H.W. Bush and think that he had so many advantages that we don't.

While there may be some truth to that, we neglect to realize that his (and others like him) life was anything but easy and he suffered plenty. At 21 years old he was shot down from an airplane over the Pacific during World War II. He saw close friends perish. A few years later he watched his first daughter suffer and die from leukemia at the tender age of three.

He didn't use these things as excuses. He had an amazing attitude, which made all the difference and allowed him to create a tremendous impact.

10 Ways to Stop Self-Sabotaging Your Goals

Now for the 10 ways in which many people self-sabotage their fitness goals followed by a discussion on how to prevent them. Some will be mindset-oriented and others will be related to technology (i.e. the things you'll do to lose weight). People tend to:

- **Self-Sabotaging Technique #1: Thinking understanding equals doing.** The reality is this book could have been written in under ten words. Let's give that a try. "Move more. Eat less." Wow, only four words. I wonder if that could be a best seller. Many people have good intentions and even make a plan but they fail to follow through. They don't truly understand something unless they implement it. In reality, it's not head knowledge you're after. It's behavioral change.

- **Self-Sabotaging Technique #2: Giving will power too much credit.** While you will certainly have to exercise self-control to a certain extent, successful people don't give themselves too much credit. I have a friend who is in a business where unfortunately infidelity is not uncommon. He maintains a successful career and has a great family life. When I asked him how he stays on the straight and narrow, he said something simple but profound: "I stay away from the after-hour events. I just go home to my family. I know if I remove myself from those situations, I'll be less tempted to make a foolish decision." In many cases it isn't about will power—it's about being mindful about setting yourself up for success and avoiding situations that will cause you to choose unwisely.

- **Self-Sabotaging Technique #3: Not wanting it bad enough.** Achieving a positive physical change is hard. It will require sacrifice. You won't be prepared to make those sacrifices if you don't have a "burning desire" to achieve the goal.

  The pain associated with change, any change, is very real.

  It hurts to eat right and exercise. It hurts, especially when there doesn't seem to be an immediate benefit. There is pain from sore muscles. There is pain in planning and preparing for healthy eating. It might mean less time comfortably relaxing in front of the tube. And you can't just make one good choice. Hitting the gym after work but then rewarding yourself with a bowl of ice cream won't get you very far.

  Some people try to use imagery when attempting positive change. Imagery is certainly a valuable tool. But when it comes down to the real pain associated with change and the imaginary pleasure, too often the latter will lose. That's because we can feel the pain now (e.g. muscle soreness) but we can't see the long-term result (e.g. weight loss, a healthier life, etc.) just yet.

  What can one do about this dilemma?

  You'll need to make the pleasure as real as the pain. The good news is that right decisions lead to good feelings which lead to more right decisions. More right decisions lead to results. And that's what you're after.

Here are three things you can do stay on the straight and narrow.

First, celebrate small victories. This could be little rewards equal in magnitude to the tasks completed. Sometimes completing a task is a reward in itself. You can get pleasure from constantly pushing yourself to achieve more.

Next, write goals down. There is power in putting pen to paper. It brings clarity. A list of tasks can keep you focused on what's important. Without a list people risk becoming a "wandering generality." A "wandering generality" is someone who isn't specific in where they're going and will probably not end up in a desirable place.

Finally, get accountability. You have to realize that the help of others can catapult you much further than you can go on your own. Have someone help or coach you through your change. This can be a paid coach, a friend, or a family member. I have wanted to write a book for years, but it didn't come to fruition until I hired a writing coach for support, guidance, and accountability.

Change is certainly not easy. I can assure you that anyone who thinks it is hasn't achieved anything significant. Change involves pain. Change involves sacrifice. The good news is that with each step of the way your character is developed, which is the greatest reward of all.

- **Self-Sabotaging Technique #4: Thinking you don't need help**. This one might be difficult to hear, but if you think you are above people that need help, guidance, and accountability then you may be lacking an essential ingredient for physical change—humility. In general, people are very poor at taking responsibility or even being accurate in their assessment of themselves. Studies show that when people are asked to give a report of how many calories they consumed in a day, they are up to 60% off. Acknowledging your shortcomings and seeking guidance and accountability from others can go a long way to helping you reach your fitness and weight loss goals.

- **Self-Sabotaging Technique #5: Thinking everything will go smoothly.** Here are some of the flawed beliefs and pitfalls people fall into. They think:

  o **Enthusiasm won't fade** – Everyone starts off gung ho. That initial excitement fades and you'll need to have a plan to keep going when the going gets tough.

  o **It will be smooth sailing once they've reached the goal** – Achieving a goal is hard but sustaining success is even more difficult. You will still need to do the work once you hit your target. Of course, it's more than worth it!

  o **Nothing unexpected will occur** – Life happens. Kids get sick. You'll suffer minor injuries. You may not always get the sleep you need to feel your best. What are you going to do when these things happen?

  o **The perceived benefits will equal their effort** – This one is extremely common. People feel like they deserve some sort of reward for their efforts. Maybe it took 10 years to put the weight on but if they exercise every day for a week they feel like they deserve to drop 20 pounds. When that doesn't happen they get frustrated. There are many factors when it comes to weight loss and nothing is guaranteed. The one reward you can count on is what the process of trying does to you. It'll make you a better person and that in and of itself is the greatest reward.

- **Self-Sabotaging Technique #6: Not letting yourself get uncomfortable**. Many times, we simply aren't challenging ourselves enough. Moderate exercise is great but we need to make ourselves uncomfortable both physically and mentally at times. Our muscles, heart, brain need to be pushed a little more than they're used to in order to grow.

- **Self-Sabotaging Technique #7: Not doing the things you know you need to do whether you feel like it or not.** Do you ever wish there was more time in the day so you could get the important things done such as exercise, preparing healthy meals, etc.? If so, you're not alone.

  The reality is everyone has the same amount of time each day. In general, people that prioritize certain things don't have more time than others. They simply make time. They've learned to manage themselves, and most importantly, to execute!

  No matter how busy you think you are, there are people that are "busier" getting it done. I had a client early on in my training career named Paul. He had four kids under seven years old and a busy accounting firm, but he got up each day at 5 a.m. to get his workout in. I know another great guy, Rich, who is a town supervisor and is as "busy" as they come. Regardless, he's in the gym regularly whether it's 5 a.m. or 4 p.m.

- **Self-Sabotaging Technique #8: Using ineffective technologies.** If I told you that you could become a millionaire by sleeping as much as possible and spending every penny you get, you'd look at me like I was crazy. But that's exactly what people often do with their fitness programs. They try with things that will never work. Things like doing only aerobic exercise or depriving themselves of much needed nutrients for extended periods of time.

- **Self-Sabotaging Technique #9: Missing important puzzle pieces.** Fitness is like one gigantic puzzle. You'll need to include all the pieces to make it work. Some people are really good in one area but others are severely lacking in another. All of the following need to be addressed for optimal health.

  o   Effective nutrition

  o   Progressive resistance training program

  o   Some aerobic activity

  o   Proper sleep

  o   Stress management

  o   Effective supplementation

- **Self-Sabotaging Technique #10: Trying to do too much.** People set themselves up for failure when they attempt huge overhauls. Instead of trying to get up two hours earlier, how about just 10 minutes at a time? How about just one extra glass of water per day? Or just one additional day of exercise?

Asking the Right Questions

Another habit that will lead to your success is self-reflection. A technique I've been using with myself and some coaching clients is asking some basic questions each day. These aren't just any questions. They should…

- **Be answered with a yes/no or a number. Something quantifiable**. For example, "How did I do today?" wouldn't work but "Did I exercise today?" would.

- **Only take about two minutes.** For that reason I recommend just 4-6 questions to start.

- **Be personal.** In other words, I can't give you your questions.

They have to be things that make sense to you and your values. They also should be things you need accountability on. If you always have a healthy breakfast that probably doesn't have to be on the list.

*Bonus – You don't always have control over the outcome but you can always control your effort. For that reason, I recommend using the word "try" in your questions. Here are some examples that I've used myself or with coaching clients.

How hard did I try, on a scale of 1-10, to…

- Get a good night's sleep

- Exercise

- Avoid late night snacking

- Drink water throughout the day

- Take my vitamins

- Set goals for myself

*I learned about these self-reflection questions from Marshall Goldsmith in his book, *Triggers,* and adapted them to fitness.

Common Traits of Those Who Successfully Lose Weight

While there are usually several ways to do things, science and my experience point to three things that successful weight losers have in common.

1. **Exercise** – People that lose weight and keep it off do some kind of exercise most days of the week.

2. **Breakfast** – Highly fit people make it a habit to start their day with a well-balanced breakfast.

3. **Journaling** – This one takes some self-discipline but is extremely powerful.

It really is that simple! Schedule your exercise in, eat a balanced breakfast, and write down what foods you are putting in your body so that you are mindful of what you eat and you don't over-consume calories. You can do this!

Top Seven Habits of Successful People

For fun, I want to add in this list of the seven habits I've noticed successful people tend to have. I've studied the habits of the fittest people for years. Oftentimes, these people are also very successful in other areas of their lives. Check out the list of the top 7 Habits of Successful people that I've compiled after years of research, especially #3.

1. **Gratitude** – The most successful people practice some sort of gratitude. Some literally make a list of 5 things they are thankful for each morning. Best-selling author of *The 4-Hour Work Week*, Tim Ferris, does this. I also know Oprah is a fan of this practice.

2. **Quiet time** – Some just sit quietly. Some pray. Others meditate. Either way, the highest achievers generally practice some sort of quiet time upon waking. This helps prevent them from jumping right into reaction mode first thing in the morning.

3. **They make their bed** – This might come as a surprise to you. Here's why it's true. Starting off your day by making the bed gives you a quick win, an accomplishment. This sets the tone for more accomplishments. There's also the idea that how people do the little things is how they'll do the bigger things. And as Navy Seal Adm. William McRaven said in his amazing commencement speech at the University of Texas, "…and if by chance you have a miserable day, you will come home to a bed that is made."

4. **Breakfast** – Starting the day with a healthy breakfast will give you the energy you need for a positive and productive day. A couple of my favorite breakfast options are eggs and veggies, oatmeal with protein powder, or a healthy smoothie

with high quality protein.

5. **Guzzle water** – Do you have trouble getting enough water in? Try what high achievers know. Drinking a glass or two of water first thing in the morning helps ensure you remain hydrated. A lack of water is one of the most common reasons for fatigue and lack of focus. And just like making the bed, it'll give you a quick win. Start the day by chugging some water and sip throughout the day. I personally don't allow myself any coffee or tea in the morning until I put down a solid 32 ounces of clean water!

6. **Exercise** – You know this had to be on the list. If possible get some exercise in the morning. It will help keep you focused. Breaking a sweat in the AM will leave you with a tremendous feeling of accomplishment. If you can't always train in the AM, no worries. I don't always, myself. Just do it when you can (e.g. weekends), but make sure you get at least two strength training sessions in per week, regardless of what time they are.

7. **Make a list** – Successful people run their day. They don't let their day run them. Making a list related to your goals and checking off the tasks is a sure fire way to get from where you are to where you want to be.

8. **Multi-vitamin** – I know it's supposed to be 7 habits but I wanted to "go the extra mile." Taking a multi-vitamin each morning is an easy way to ensure you are getting the nutrients you need. It's just that, an insurance policy.

CHAPTER 5:

OVERCOMING PROCRASTINATION

IN ALL AREAS, the people who are successful are action takers. Being passive won't get the job done. In this chapter you'll learn practical ways to make sure you are in the habit of getting the right things done.

"Nothing comes merely by thinking about it."
– John Wanamaker

Procrastination is perhaps the biggest obstacle when it comes to getting things done. In this chapter I'll discuss why people put things off and more importantly how you can beat procrastination once and for all.

One of the main reasons for procrastination is that there are usually no immediate negative consequences from not doing important habits. For example, if you skip one workout and eat a doughnut, nothing noticeable will happen. It's after extended periods of time of skipping workouts and eating doughnuts that obesity and heart attacks happen. People have a hard time seeing into the future and being long-term minded. Instead, you need to realize the immediate positives (e.g. feeling accomplished).

Action Steps

Procrastination is something everyone struggles with to a certain extent and in certain areas. Here are two things you can do to overcome it and make progress.

1. **Set an appointment** – When you have a doctor's appointment, you make it a point to get there. You can do the same thing with your workout and/or other healthy habits.

2. **Execute** – While people often start out motivated, once they take action they start to build momentum, which is a beautiful thing. I don't think I've ever heard someone say they regretted doing a workout.

Recognizing that you're procrastinating is the first step to making a change. Knowing you should do something isn't enough. It's executing that counts!

*Perhaps you are completely dialed in with your nutrition and workouts. If that's the case, props to you, but maybe these ideas apply to other areas? Career. Finances. Relationships. It's all important. If one wheel falls off, it affects the rest.

More on Procrastination

The word procrastination has an interesting meaning. The Latin *pro* means "toward" and *crastinus* means "tomorrow." After all, who can say that they aren't guilty of "putting off till tomorrow"?

I think I figured out why people procrastinate. They don't want to do what they know they have to do.

Seriously, there are several reasons why people procrastinate. I'll share one reason why I have in the past. I lacked confidence in my ability. I didn't think I could succeed and didn't want to prove that by trying. I, of course, didn't realize that at the time. This was true in my school example earlier.

Other reasons people procrastinate include not thinking the task is worth it (Will going out for a run really make a difference?) and following the path of least resistance (Should I get up and get to the gym or watch this show?).

Many techniques are used for putting things off. Here are some that are commonly used by people.

- Reward themselves before doing what they probably won't get around to doing. Ever tell yourself this? "Once I get a good night's rest, I'll get up and exercise."

- Estimate the time they have and decide it's not enough. For example, they say, "I only have 15 minutes so there's no point in doing it because I need 30 minutes." One of our team members admitted to this one.

- They think (and sometimes talk) about all the things they want to do but never actually do them. This fantasy land provides immediate enjoyment but never leads to real results.

There are other techniques that are used. People seem to be quite sophisticated in procrastination. But I'd rather focus on what you CAN do about it. Here are three in addition to the ones already mentioned…

1. **Reward yourself only after a difficult task, not before** – For example, "I'll allow myself one treat only if I eat effectively for the rest of the day/week." Even better, reward yourself with a non-food item (e.g. movie tickets).

2. **Take responsibility for excuses** – If you only have 10 minutes to do something, recognize that you'll have 10 minutes less to do when finishing it later.

3. **Set a deadline** – This can be difficult because you know the deadline is something arbitrary that you are setting. However, what would happen if you had to give $300 to a cause you despised if you didn't finish your task by a certain date?

Here's another point that I think deserves more attention.

Confront the Brutal Facts

Expect obstacles and difficulties. Remaining optimistic is important when you need to persevere in order to reach a goal but it's only half the picture. The other half is being realistic about the brutal realities. I've read many stories of people overcoming unimaginable circumstances (e.g. being held in a prisoner of war camp for years). The ones who survive have faith but they also acknowledge the reality they're in. They don't ignore the facts.

Take for instance our client Dina. Dina was moving along doing all the right things in her quest to improve her health and fitness. Then out of nowhere she was diagnosed with an aggressive form of breast cancer. I can't even imagine how difficult this must have been. How did Dina respond? Did she crawl up in a corner and give up? I wouldn't have blamed her if she did but she absolutely didn't! Did she ignore the reality that she had an extremely difficult road ahead of her? No, she didn't do that either. She had faith that she would overcome the cancer but she knew it wouldn't be easy. In fact, check out this message she posted in our private Facebook group after she was diagnosed:

"I just wanted my TBBC Family to know that I was recently diagnosed with an aggressive form of breast cancer called invasive ductal carcinoma (her2+). I have to go through 2 rounds of chemo and then a double mastectomy. After surgery I will need to be on 2 more drugs for a year & possibly radiation....the prognosis is good but there are no guarantees in life...I know it's hard for people not to share so I don't mind sharing my story...I am a fighter but I have an up-hill battle in front of me & I will make it to the top...I will see you all at the gym."

Do you see how she has a perfect blend of faith while not ignoring her reality? She has a difficult road ahead of her and is determined to win. I'm proud to say that Dina is doing great and still showing up to all of her sessions while she endures the treatment.

I hope you never have to go through something this difficult but the reality is there will be some obstacles and difficulties. Even smaller obstacles like a kid getting the sniffles can throw you off. This is why it's important not to ignore this concept.

Rather than ignore problems and obstacles, meet them head on. Successful people aren't people with no problems. They're people that find solutions and act on them.

Some people make excuses and when things aren't urgent enough they put them off. Maybe you fall into this category. What you want to do is find a way to make them more meaningful. Once you find out what will make the goal stick, you'll do what it takes to achieve that goal. For some it might mean getting up early to work out or skipping the cake at a party. This can only happen once the goal is a priority, not just a wish.

At the end of the day it's all about ACTION and an action-oriented mindset. You must stop talking about it and start doing it. Do it. And do it. And do it.

There is never a "perfect time." For some reason, people always want to start on Monday or even worse New Years. There is no need to wait any longer. It's time! Let go of all the reasons why you can't or think you aren't good enough. You are good enough right now and you can do it. Even if you have a large goal, break it up into manageable pieces. You still have time. Don't give up. You can do it. I believe in you.

Now go out there and do the thing you know you need to do!

CHAPTER 6:

PRIORITIZING FAMILY AND FITNESS

THERE IS NO doubt that life gets busy. You might have a family, a career, and friends. Fitting fitness into the other areas of your life may not be easy but it's worth it. In this chapter I'll show you how.

> *"I've learned that you can't have everything*
> *and do everything at the same time."*
> **– Oprah Winfrey**

When I first met Claudine she was stressed out. She had a husband and five kids, a career, and a mortgage. I met Claudine at a party. A mutual friend of ours was also a client. Claudine explained that she wanted to lose weight but time was her biggest obstacle. She was so busy taking care of everyone else. When would she have time for self-care?

*Check out Claudines's transformation (including 60 pounds of weight loss) as well as other client showcases by going to www.lifitnessbootcamp.com and clicking on "SUCCESS STORIES."

Putting Your Own Mask on First

I've been traveling to Kentucky every few months to work with a coach. Yes I have a coach. If I didn't, wouldn't I be a hypocrite? After all, I'm always preaching the benefits of having a coach. If I'm not willing to invest in a coach, why should I expect anyone else to?

My airline of choice has been Southwest. The main reason I started using them is because of convenience (they fly out of Islip, NY). This way Melissa can drive me to the airport if scheduling permits. If not, it's super easy to park my car there.

I've learned some great business lessons from Southwest...

- **They make doing business easy.** When I had to change my flight with enough notice it was as smooth as could be. I didn't have to jump through a whole bunch of hurdles.

- **They keep things simple**. Each time I've flown with them, it's been the same type of plane. This keeps my costs down which I appreciate. This is partly why we don't offer massage, yoga, Pilates, or a smoothie bar at our fitness facilities. We specialize in small group and team training.

- **They're fun**. This is one of TBBC's core values. I always get a chuckle from Southwest's silly announcements. Flying is not always the most pleasurable thing (kind of like working out) so anything that makes it more fun is appreciated.

I can't help but think when I hear the announcement about putting your own mask on first. You know, the one that goes something like this: "In the unlikely event that cabin pressure drops, secure your own mask before helping others."

Fortunately, I've never had to use the oxygen mask on a plane. I hope you haven't either. But why do they advise us to do this? It's because you can't possibly help others if you aren't safe yourself.

While most people get this concept in a life or death situation, they often neglect it in their day to day.

Yes, life gets hectic. It's not easy, but you must put your own mask on first if you want to be effective.

I'm a better husband and father when I exercise, pray, think, and read.

I'm a better leader for my team and our Warriors when I do those things as well. Would you want to invest in a coach who you knew didn't prioritize their own health and fitness to some degree? Sorry to judge, but it's amazing how many chubby fitness professionals I see. Some of them don't even work out! One that I knew regularly ate McDonalds for lunch and smoked cigarettes.

My wife feels the same way as I do about taking care of herself. With two small children, it's a challenge for Melissa to put her mask on first but when she does, we're all better for it.

It's not always going to be perfect but there will be a direct correlation between taking care of yourself and your effectiveness as a spouse, parent, friend, co-worker, etc.

Here are some areas to check...

- How much sleep are you getting?

- Are you being coached on your fitness at some level?

- Who's holding you accountable?

- Are you eating a healthy breakfast each day?

- Do you take some time during the day to de-stress, even if it's just a few minutes?

If these things are neglected for too long, they will result in some sort of problem. Be proactive. Put your own mask on, and you'll be better for it.

Talk is cheap. People say certain things are important to them but their actions don't back it up. This is extremely common in the business world. A CEO will say that his family means everything to him, but then he barely knows the middle names of his children because he's working 16-hour days to "provide" for them.

Calendars and Checkbooks Don't Lie

Do people still use checkbooks? If not I guess we can change the above to "Calendars and bank statements" don't lie. The point is if you look at how you spend your time (i.e. calendar) and money (i.e. bank statement), you can see where your values lie. You can say your health is important but if exercise and wellness visits are nowhere to be found on your calendar, I think you need to re-evaluate things.

Is your health and fitness really important to you? Does your calendar reflect that?

Spend some time writing down your values. Values are essentially what's important to you. Here are some of mine…

- Reading

- Fitness

- Family

- Church

- Brazilian Jiu-Jitsu

- Developing relationships

I suggest using your values to create qualifiers in decision-making. What I mean by this is when you are making a decision throughout the day, ask yourself, "Does this match up with what I say is important to me?" Using the health/fitness example, you may decide to skip going out for wings and drinks since it doesn't align with your value of fitness.

Since you have other people in your life that count on you, it helps to communicate your values with them. Melissa is very aware that fitness is important to me. I'm also aware of her values. This helps us support each other in our decision-making. Go ahead and share your values with those that are important to you.

If It's Not a YES, It's a No

Remember also that you need to have boundaries. Your time is one of the most valuable thing that you have. And it will never come back. Everyone has 24 hours in their day and decides what they do with many of those hours. You need to respect yourself enough to have limits. Everyone has a capacity. The problem is many people are running too close or over that limit. Boundaries aren't just about saying no; they are about saying YES to what's more important to you. Every time you say yes to one thing, you're saying no to something else.

Pastor and author Andy Stanley says, "The difference between successful people and very successful people is that very successful people are always saying no."

What things do you need to say NO to in order to say YES to what matters most?

I'll also add that whatever you do, be all in. This means when you're working out, get after it. When you're talking to someone, be completely dialed in. When you're working, roll up your sleeves and get dirty. One percent better every day, baby!

Dating Our Cell Phones?

I was at a restaurant with my family. I couldn't help but notice a couple next to us. They had to be in their mid-twenties. They sat down, ordered drinks, and pulled out their cell phones. The guy had his head buried in his cell phone scrolling through messages that came across the top of the screen. The young lady was mostly staring off into space. How sad, I thought, that this couple can't even have a conversation with each other while on a date.

After we finished eating I went to the bathroom and noticed the guy going to the bathroom, while on his cell phone! (Sorry for the visual.) When I returned to the table, the girl was now on her cell phone scrolling through Facebook. I took a look around and noticed that a solid 50 percent of the patrons were on their phones.

Caught in the Act

Then again, perhaps my wife and I are no better.

It's crazy how perceptive kids can be. My wife and I both had an eye opening experience with Alyssa, who was four at the time.

Alyssa, like most kids, loves to watch TV. Every morning we do a little reading with her but then it's a snack, juice, vitamin, and cartoons. One day, Melissa left her in front of the tube a little longer than usual so she could get some things done. Her jaw almost dropped to the floor when Alyssa asked her if she could turn the thing off! She was getting sick of it. Ouch!

I had a similar experience. One day I was working from home and had my phone off for much of the day. When I finished working, I came out of my office but was checking my phone as Alyssa was trying to tell me something. Then she paused and said, "Dad, you read a lot. You read books. You read from the computer. Even now you're reading from your phone." Ridden with guilt, I shut my phone off and pulled her towards me. Realizing she'll only be four once, I told her, "Sweetie, nothing on that phone is more important than you. From now on when I'm with you the phone stays off." She smiled.

We now have a family rule that the phones go away during family time, especially when we're eating together.

Whether you have kids or not, cell phones and other technology can be extremely distracting. Here are some tips to prevent technology winning your attention at the expense of the things that matter most. These are just ideas. Do what works for you.

- **Use the good aspects of technology but avoid the bad.** If there is an app that is useful to you, go ahead and use it. Just don't let it be an excuse to surf Facebook for three hours.

- **No e-mail or Facebook in the morning**. Have you ever noticed that when you start your day looking at your phone, you immediately get sucked into reaction mode? I want you telling your day where to go, not the other way around. I've been waiting until 12:30 p.m. to check e-mail or Facebook most days and I can't tell you how much better I feel.

- **Schedule your time**. If you enjoy surfing Facebook, go for it. Set a timer for 10 minutes and surf away but when that timer goes off, shut it down.

- **Take e-mail off your phone**. I did this and I get a lot of e-mails. You can do it too.

- **Don't check e-mails you're not prepared to respond to.**

This one has been huge for me. In the past I would check e-mails knowing I couldn't respond until later. Then I would think about them all day and waste precious energy. What's worse is I would sometimes lack the control to wait and I would send a rushed response.

When I first started taking some of these steps, I was worried people wouldn't understand. At the end of the day, you have to teach people how to communicate with you. The people that matter most in my life know that I'm probably not going to answer an e-mail or a text on Sunday. That's family time.

The same thing goes when it comes to weight loss for busy people. Turn your phone off or on silent when you're working out. That's your time. Enjoy it and make the most of it. Let the people who are important to you know your workout schedule and hopefully they'll support your effort.

How to Raise Fit Kids

I was driving my wife and daughter home from Grandma in Pennsylvania's house when Alyssa (three years old at the time) opened up her snack, rolled down the window and sent her wrapper flying out the window. "Am I raising a kid with no concern for the environment?" I thought. Before letting my anger get the best of me, I calmly asked, "Sweetie, why did you do that?" Without missing a beat she said, "But Daddy, you threw an apple out of the window one time." I thought for a second. She was right. I had tossed an apple out of the window about a week prior. It was my fault that my three-year-old had littered. While the apple is biodegradable, she wouldn't understand that. It's not a good excuse anyway.

Before I had kids I thought it was crazy how people seem to have such similar mannerisms as their parents. I remember standing in line somewhere when I was in my twenties and I realized that I was standing with my hands folded the same way my dad would. It kind of freaked me out. Now that I have children of my own, it's very clear. I see them studying my wife and me. This is where they get the majority of their info. Powerful stuff.

This concept certainly applies to fitness and nutrition as well. In fact, check out this statistic. A child with just one obese parent has a 50% chance of being obese. A child with two obese parents has an 80% risk.

We try to incorporate "exercise" into our everyday life. We go for walks, play at the park, have races, wrestle, etc. Sometimes we actually work out together. We always make it fun and include some kind of game or competition. These are my goals:

1. Move

2. Have fun

3. Use it as a teachable moment

One time we went to a park and did a modified conditioning workout we do at TBBC.

The warm-up included jumping jacks, squats, tag, and "races."

For the workout we all chose one exercise plus we all agreed on a fourth exercise. We would run back and forth on the playground doing ten repetitions of any of the four exercises. I chose dips. Melissa chose squats. Alyssa chose an exercise that she made up which resembled a cross between an iron cross (going into a squat position with arms out) and star jump (crouching down into a squat and then jumping while opening the arms). The fourth exercise was a basic jump. The goal was to go for 15 minutes.

We had so much fun. About half way through, Alyssa wanted to stop and go on the swing. She did and that was fine. I want her to enjoy playing. It's not so important for her to be structured right now. I continued the workout and added in some other exercises including tricep extensions off the bench and pull-ups from a tree branch. At one point Alyssa looked up from the swing while I was doing pull-ups and said, "I wish I could do that someday." I have no doubt that she will.

Ask yourself this question:

How can I incorporate healthy habits into my home life this week? I'd love to know what you come up with.

CHAPTER 7:

FINDING THE RIGHT FITNESS PROGRAM FOR YOU

ONE OF THE main reasons people don't stick with a fitness program is due to boredom. In this chapter I'll discuss ways to keep your program fresh and exciting. Find out how to make boredom with exercise or your fitness routine a thing of the past.

"Don't live the same year 75 times and call it a life."
— Robin Sharma

Now we get to more of the nuts and bolts of the program. It seems like everyone's looking for the magic program, the one that works better than all the others. The best program for you is the program that you'll stick with. It's that simple. It's ironic that many of the folks that argue over which program is best aren't consistently doing any program. They're wasting their time dissing other programs. While there are certainly better ways of doing things, any program can have benefits. You just have to do it.

After helping people lose fat for almost 20 years, my team and I have developed a program that burns fat and builds strength you can use. All while having fun!

There are several programs that work and you'll have to choose which one is best for you.

The bottom line is you have to move.

With that said, if you're looking for a program with a proven track record, feel free to set up a "Success in Fitness" Strategy Session with us. I'd love to meet and chat with you and see if we might be a good fit to work together. You can set that up by going to www. lifitnessbootcamp.com and clicking "CONTACT."

This is the next step you'll want to take to begin your transformation.

Whatever it is you decide to do, here are some things to take into consideration.

- **Make sure you enjoy it** – While you probably won't like every aspect of your fitness program (most people don't enjoy being uncomfortable), there should be something enjoyable about it. Maybe you like a certain aspect of it or how you feel after. Perhaps you like the people you train with or your coach.

- **Make sure it's safe** – Safety must come first. That's the #1 rule at our facility: don't hurt anyone! If you're hurt you're not making progress. Be sure that safety is of the utmost concern in whatever program you choose. Unfortunately some facilities and coaches (if we can call them that) just want to push you to the limit even if you sacrifice your technique. This is also why I'm not a huge fan of fitness videos. While they certainly have their place, you're not getting feedback. What if you're doing it wrong but have no idea? To me it's just not worth it.

- **Make sure it works for you** – It must be as convenient as possible. If you're driving 30 minutes to go train, it's only a matter of time before excuses start popping up. It also must work with your schedule. If you are someone (like me) who doesn't have the greatest energy in the evening, make sure you schedule your workouts before work.

Incorporating Fitness into Daily Life

It is important to have a fitness routine, but it is also important just to make it a point to *get off your butt*. People sit entirely too much. Many people have a daily routine like this...

- Wake up

- Get ready

- **Sit** and have breakfast

- **Sit** in the car and drive to work

- Get to work and **sit** while working at a computer

- **Sit** in the car and drive home

- Do a few things around the house

- **Sit** down to have dinner

- **Sit** on the couch and watch TV

- Get ready for bed

- Sleep 5-8 hours

- Repeat

As you can see, sitting is a major problem. Too much of it can lead to...

- **A bad back** – Sitting causes muscles to tighten. What's more, poor sitting posture can wreak havoc on your vertebrae.

- **Chronic disease** – Even people who work out and/or aren't fat need to move throughout the day. If they don't, physiological changes can occur that may lead to some terrible health problems.

- **Weight gain** – This one should be obvious. We, as a nation, are becoming more and more sedentary. Besides all the driving and computer time, everything is instant and easy for us. We have remote controls (so we don't even have to get up from the couch), microwave dinners, and fast food (so we don't even have to expend energy preparing food). We even have dishwashers to clean our dishes for us. All of these conveniences come with a price. They are adding to the increasing problem of obesity.

Now that we've identified the problem inherent in too much sitting, let's discuss some things you can do about it…

- **Be careful where you park** – Have you ever circled around a parking lot for 10 minutes just to find a spot that was a few feet closer? I'm sure you haven't, but maybe you know someone who has? I suggest doing the opposite—intentionally park further away to get some extra activity. It will require a shift in thinking, but those extra steps add up. If you want to be different than most people (i.e. healthier), you'll have to start doing things differently than most people.

- **Little things add up** – Perhaps the thought of exercising an hour plus per day is overwhelming. I get it. How about 30 minutes per day then? I'm sure you can make that work. If you did that just 5 days per week, you'd be getting 2.5 hours of exercise per week. If 30 minutes seems like a lot now, start with 20. Or 10. Or 5. Or even 2. I'm really trying to drive home the point that something is better than nothing and little things add up.

- **Set an alarm** – Now that Total Body has grown, I find myself becoming more sedentary. Where I used to spend most of my time on the floor coaching clients, I'm now spending more and more time on "back end" stuff. For example, right now I'm sitting as I type this. What I've started to do is set a timer anywhere from 25-45 minutes to get some focused work done. Once that timer goes off, I try to stop what I'm doing for 5-10 minutes and do some moving around. I might go for a 5-minute walk. I may stretch or even do some calisthenics. This gets my legs working again and keeps me focused. Don't underestimate the importance of little things like this. They can improve…

o **Cholesterol** – While your body makes cholesterol and a certain amount is normal for healthy function, too much of it can pose problems.

o **Body Mass Index (BMI)** – BMI is a measure of body fat based on your weight in relation to your height. Generally, higher BMI scores are correlated with certain diseases (e.g. heart disease and diabetes).

o **Glucose tolerance** – This is the body's ability to use the sugar glucose and is used to test for diabetes and pre-diabetes.

o **Waist circumference** – Waist circumference is a practical tool to test for abdominal fat and chronic disease risk.

Principles of a Successful Fitness Program

While I mentioned there are several exercise programs you can choose from, there are some main principles we apply with our program that I recommend finding for yourself. You want a fitness program that…

1. Has a dynamic warm-up – A proper warm-up doesn't have to take a long time and it will get your body ready for the activity you'll be doing. This will result in more efficiency and better results. You'll also improve coordination that will help prevent injury and perhaps most important, you'll be completely dialed in mentally. A more focused training session equals more fat loss!

A dynamic warm-up is a series of movements designed not only to increase body temperature but also to activate the nervous system (think of this as the connection from the brain to the body), improve range of motion (this will make you more limber), and correct any asymmetries or imbalances (e.g. perhaps one side is tighter than the other).

The days of just doing a quick 5-minute walk to warm up are long gone. We now know several reasons for a proper warm up.

- **Injury prevention** – Warming up and strengthening areas that are more prone to injury will help keep you healthy. Certain exercises promote joint integrity. Your joints support bones and the better they can do this the safer and more efficient you'll be.

- **Flexibility** – Certain movements (e.g. twisting to get something) put your body in compromised positions. A proper flexibility program will allow speed and precision during movement as well as develop proper motor patterns (how your brain relates to muscles).

- **Core stability** – Almost all of your movement requires some level of abdominal activation (the muscles in your stomach being turned on) and control of torso position while the limbs are moving through space. Core stability training will allow you to do these movements more safely and more efficiently, which will also allow you to burn more fat with your program!

2. Makes fitness FUN – You'll want to strive to make the training fun. You can do that by…

- **Partner sessions** – Working together with a partner adds so much fun. Not only does this provide some extra accountability but you'll have a blast!

- **Training as a team** – Theoretically, you can have anywhere from 2 to 8 or even 20 people training together. For many people, the days of playing together on a team are long gone, but you can still get that feeling by training as a group. Not all of the sessions have to be this way but even once or twice per week or month adds a nice touch!

- **Planned challenges** – I like to add enjoyment to my sessions by including timed challenges. For example, you might perform a certain number of repetitions as fast as possible or perform as much "work" as possible in a given time period. If you're wired with a competitive edge, this can make the time go much faster.

- **Music** – You'll want to match the music to your training session. It's amazing what the right tune at the right time can do to the energy and motivation of the room!

- **Shorter workouts** – You might consider intentionally adding brief sessions throughout the week. Not every session has to be a marathon.

- **Do what you like** – Try to incorporate what you like. Some feel empowered by slamming medicine balls and oversized ropes into the floor. Others enjoy boxing workouts. Add the activities you enjoy. It's also OK to skip things you're dreading periodically. While I think it's important and necessary to do things you don't like, sometimes it's just one of those days and that's OK.

- **Get outside** – There's nothing like being one with nature as you exercise. Take your sessions on the road. Go to a nearby park or right outside your front door and breathe the fresh air.

- **Track progress** – This theme is coming up a lot in this book. There's a reason for it. Goals can motivate you. As you see yourself moving closer to the target, you'll embrace the process.

- **Learn something new** – Incorporating different movements into your training sessions keeps things fresh. This way you're learning something new and getting into great shape. One of the biggest recent breakthroughs in exercise research is what working out does for our brains. This is one of the greatest benefits. Exercise actually creates new brain cells.

- **Mix it up** – Most people LOVE variety. For that reason, strive to make each session just a little different, even if it's just switching the order of the exercises.

3. Doesn't neglect muscle – One of the biggest reasons our clients succeed with us is because we make sure they have a concern for muscle.

Regina, a 50-year-old saleswoman with a busy schedule, came to us looking to tone up. When she realized she would be doing resistance training (i.e. lifting weights) with us, she became very skeptical. In the past she had done different diets and mostly aerobic activity which led her to the yo-yo effect. Sometimes she'd be up. Sometimes she'd be down. At the point when she came to our facility she was up. I assured her that the resistance training we would be doing would help her with her goals of "toning."

Thankfully Regina trusted us, because she's down 18 pounds in just a few short months. She was also able to come off blood pressure and cholesterol medication.

What Regina didn't know before she came in was that women don't have the natural hormones to build the freakish muscles they fear. To drive home the point, many 18-year-old boys struggle to build muscle. Meanwhile they may have up to 10 times the testosterone as women!

As people age they naturally lose muscle tissue. This is problematic because muscle is needed to burn fat. The less muscle you have, the less fat you can burn. Metabolism slows.

You'll want to do everything you can to keep the muscle you have. Muscle is the physical location where fat is burned.

Any exercise or nutrition program that ignores muscle should be avoided like the plague!

4. Improves Your Life

This is an important principle to a successful fitness program. This section is about what most people really want. Of course, many people desire weight loss but there's more to it.

The deeper goal most people have is they want to get more out of life. They want to live life how it's meant to be lived. And it's meant to be enjoyed.

For that reason it's important to do a program that not only helps you lose weight but helps you...

- **Develop the strength you need to perform your daily tasks and then some** – This includes movements and activities that are at least somewhat related to what you do in your everyday life.

- **Stay free of injury** – It's hard to make progress if you're injured!

- **Improve your endurance** – More endurance will not only make you healthier but it will also improve your mental fortitude as well as your self-confidence.

- **Develop mental fortitude** – This can transfer to other areas of your life. If you can push through a really tough workout, that problem you have at work might not seem so daunting.

- **Feel more limber** – Improved flexibility will improve your posture, lessen aches and pains, and even help you live longer!

- **Lose body fat and get leaner** – You'll be looking and feeling your best.

- **Improve your core strength** – This is where all movement starts. A more powerful core equals a stronger you!

- **Have more energy** – This means more energy for the things you enjoy and for the people you love.

- **Develop power** – This will help you do the things you need to do more efficiently. It's also one of the first things we lose with age so it's important to maintain.

There are many other benefits people want to enjoy, but it all boils down to living life how it's meant to be lived!

CHAPTER 8:

THE MOST IMPORTANT MEAL OF THE DAY

I'M SURE YOU'VE been taught that breakfast is the most important meal of the day. In this chapter, I'll explain why and how you can start your day off on the right foot. Examples will also be provided.

> *"When you wake up in the morning, Pooh," said Piglet at last, "what's the first thing you say to yourself?"*
>
> *"What's for breakfast?" said Pooh. "What do you say, Piglet?"*
>
> *"I say, I wonder what's going to happen exciting today?" said Piglet.*
>
> *Pooh nodded thoughtfully. "It's the same thing," he said.*
> ***– A.A. Milne***

Your mother was right. You should stand up taller and you should eat breakfast. Breakfast truly is the most important meal. It sets the tone for the day. I notice with myself that if I don't have a balanced high-energy breakfast, my day just doesn't go right.

Some people have to learn the hard way. This includes me. I remember a day in high school when I got to school early and played an intense game of basketball before reporting to class. Unfortunately I had skipped breakfast that day. Soon after class started, I felt dizzy. I went to the bathroom and the next thing I remember I was staring at the ceiling. I had blacked out from a lack of fuel. I was only out for a few seconds and felt fine once I got some food in me.

These are the most common excuses we hear from people as to why they don't eat breakfast.

Common Excuse #1 – I don't have time

Skipping breakfast is one of the worst mistakes you can make when it comes to fitness and overall health. Many people think they don't have time for breakfast but I'm here to tell you that you must make time.

Even if time is limited, breakfast should be prioritized. It could be something simple or something prepared the night before. If you have just 5 minutes, perhaps you can make a smoothie or a quick bowl of oatmeal with some peanut butter. This is what weight loss for busy people is all about.

Common Excuse #2 – I'm not hungry in the morning

If this is the case, you may be eating too much at night. Here is the reality. It's good to be hungry in the morning. If you can go hours after waking up without eating, this may be a sign of a slow metabolism. The good news is that you can speed it up and train your body to be hungry (and also burn more fat) at the right times.

Another possible reason could be from a lack of movement or physical exercise. One of the benefits of a regular exercise program is that it will stimulate a healthy appetite. If you have time to do even a short workout first thing in the morning, that should trigger the routine of a healthy breakfast.

Common Excuse #3 – I don't like breakfast foods

I have a simple solution for this excuse. Eat a nontraditional breakfast. Nobody says you have to eat eggs for breakfast. Many people eat chicken, even Chinese food for breakfast. Mix it up! Since breakfast is so important, you may even be better off eating lunch or dinner (typically more calories) for breakfast and breakfast for dinner.

Most people have this backwards.

Eat Dinner for Breakfast

Meet Joe. Joe is a client of mine that came to my office because he struggled with his weight. He desperately wanted to lose 10-15 pounds. He had tried different things and was confused by his lack of progress. I did a dietary recall with him in which he presented me with his current eating plan.

It wasn't terrible, but I noticed a pattern I see with a lot of people. He didn't eat a lot of food in the early hours but he sure did later in the day. This is what I told Joe...

"I don't think the foods you're eating are a problem or even the total calories you're consuming. What I see as the problem is that the bulk of your calories are being ingested in the evening. Here's what I suggest. Continue eating the same foods and even the same quantities but simply reverse the order. In other words, eat dinner for breakfast and breakfast for dinner."

Joe decided to give this a try and within four weeks was down 10 pounds! We made a few additional tweaks and by the sixth week he was down 15.

Contrary to popular belief, a calorie isn't a calorie. Depending on the timing of your meals, they can have a dramatically different effect on you. For example, if you eat the bulk of your carbohydrates in the morning, chances are you will use some of them for energy throughout your busy day. If you eat those same carbohydrates right before bed, there is a much greater chance they will be stored as body fat rather than burned for energy.

One of the best things you can do for your nutrition is to follow this advice...

"Eat breakfast like a king, lunch like a prince, and dinner like a pauper."

This doesn't work for everybody and not all of the science is consistent. All I know is when I have people who are stuck try it, they seem to lose weight.

Recovery Breakfast and When to Cut Calories

If you're working out in the AM, a recovery breakfast is important. This would include some fluids to help you refuel. If you follow this advice, you will have more energy later in the day.

If your goal is weight loss, breakfast is the wrong time to cut calories. Studies show that people who eat breakfast tend to lose more weight and keep it off more than those who don't. If you're going to cut calories, do it at night!

Be sure to always start your day off right by fueling yourself properly.

Your "Start the Day Off Right" Action Plan

I don't believe in too many action steps because it can lead to paralysis by analysis. I'm only giving you two. You can handle that, right?

Action Step 1: Eat breakfast

I told you it was simple. Make sure you consume a meal as soon as possible after waking. This will set the tone for your day. You'll start the day with a metabolic boost (meaning you will immediately start burning more calories), and it will help prevent overeating later in the day. Ideally that breakfast would contain a lean protein, starchy carbs, and veggies. Don't worry, I will give examples below. If this whole breakfast thing is new to you, just make sure you eat something, because something is better than nothing. You will also learn more in the next chapter about different foods and their effects on you.

When we eat breakfast we are breaking a fast. In fact that's where the word comes from. When you don't eat for an extended period of time your body goes into starvation mode. Essentially, it thinks you're starving, so it holds onto all of the energy (and body fat) it can. This can be a good thing in certain survival scenarios. If you were stranded on an island somewhere without any food, this "starvation mode" would keep you alive. The problem arises when you get into this state when you're not actually starving.

If you go too many long periods without eating, your body may become good at storing fat (a bad thing) and very poor at burning fat (another bad thing). A key to avoiding this is by eating a well-balanced breakfast. Some bodybuilders I've known would set an alarm for the middle of the night so they could eat and not go into "starvation mode." This is obviously extreme behavior and I'm in no way condoning that practice. I just think it illustrates the importance of eating.

Action Step 2: Keep a food journal for 5 days

While the research is mixed and conflicting on many areas of nutrition, one thing is for sure. People who track what they eat by writing it down lose more weight and keep it off. If writing down everything you eat for the rest of your life is overwhelming, start with just 5 days. You'll be amazed by how it causes you to make better choices. Writing it down before you eat gives you a second to think twice.

Here are some other benefits to writing down what you eat:

- *More Weight Loss* – People that write down what they eat lose twice as much weight as those who don't keep any record of their food intake. Writing down what you eat gives you the personal accountability you need when you need it.

- *Nutritional Balance* – As with most areas, balance is crucial. If you're ignoring certain food groups, a nutrition journal can be a great way to detect this. For example, if you look back and see that you didn't consume any fruits or vegetables, you'll be able to improve by adding fruits and veggies to the following day's menu. It can also be satisfying to look back and see some of the great choices you made throughout the day.

- *Recognizing Food Intolerances* – I also recommend noting how you feel physically after eating. If you feel consistently bloated or nauseous after drinking milk, you could be lactose intolerant. Other intolerances, such as gluten, can also be detected this way. If you have a chronic disease such as diabetes or heart disease, journaling your nutrition becomes even more important. By doing so, you can avoid any problematic foods that may worsen your symptoms or condition.

Many people just eat because of their emotions or habits when they really don't need to. It's a great idea to also document your emotional state while eating. Perhaps you're eating out of boredom or as a stress coping mechanism. You might think you're hungry but in reality you're just eating out of habit. Also notice if you're alone or eating with company. Maybe eating lunch with a certain person increases the amount you eat drastically. Once you're armed with the information you need then you can make better choices.

Quick and Easy Breakfast Options

Here are some quick and creative breakfast ideas…

- **Yogurt** – I prefer Fage plain Greek yogurt. It is delicious and nutritious.

- **Banana** – I often consume a banana upon waking, especially if I have an early training session planned. I usually add a teaspoon of peanut butter.

- **Blended breakfast** – Anything from fruit, whey protein powder, greens, oatmeal, and almond butter, to a variety of other ingredients might go into my blender.

- **Raisins and nuts** – They can easily be taken with you if you are in a rush.

- Depending on your activity level and what your plans are on that particular day, you may consume a breakfast containing more **whole grains**, including steel cut oats, quinoa, or wheat berries.

Super Breakfast Options

While these might not be perfect examples, we don't live in a perfect world. It's all about doing better each day and being consistent over the long haul.

Option 1   High Energy Oatmeal
1 cup steel cut oats (Dry)
1 scoop whey protein
15 almonds or 1.5 tsp olive oil, flax seed oil, or fish oil
½ cup mixed organic frozen berries
Dash of stevia and or cinnamon if desired to make sweeter

Option 2   Happy Scrambled Eggs
6-8 oz Liquid Egg Whites (about 4-7 Large Eggs)
1 cup Steamed Wild or Brown Rice
½ Avocado or 1 oz shredded cheese
(All You Can Eat Extras) Veggies, Salsa, Hot Sauce, and Black Pepper

Option 3   Protein Shake
1 Scoop Whey Protein
16 oz of water, No Sugar Added Almond Milk, or No Sugar Added Soy Milk
1 TBSP Peanut or Almond Butter or Smart Balance Butter
1 Banana

Option 4   Non-Traditional Breakfast – Grilled Chicken
You can eat a non-traditional breakfast like a grilled chicken wrap on whole wheat with some spinach.

Additional Benefits to Eating Breakfast

Here are some additional benefits to eating breakfast…

- *Brain Power* – The brain requires fuel immediately upon waking. Without a proper breakfast, the brain simply can't perform its best. This means a reduced ability to…

o Focus – Being able to focus is crucial for us to succeed in any area.

o Remember things – Forgetting things can make life difficult.

o Solve problems – The ability to solve problems is another crucial skill.

o Be in a good mood – People that eat a healthy breakfast are less likely to become angry or irritated.

- *Emotional Health* – I know for my family, breakfast is a cherished time. It's an opportunity to connect and pour into my family. I'm not always home for dinner with my sometimes crazy work schedule, which makes this time even more special. In addition to the family bonding, breakfast is an excellent way to help instill healthy eating habits in our children. These are habits they'll most likely carry into adulthood. If we skip breakfast, our kids will see that it's not important to us. While we don't always have time for a super long breakfast, something is better than nothing.

As you can see, there are numerous benefits to starting your day with a healthy breakfast. Many people either skip or have an unhealthy breakfast. This is partly due to the hyper-paced culture in which we live. People seem to constantly be on the go. Even with all the hustle and bustle you can still make healthy choices for breakfast. Doing so will improve not only your physical health but your mental and emotional health as well; and that's one of the best investments you can make!

Hopefully I've convinced you to start your day off right, with an effective meal!

CHAPTER 9:

A SIMPLE PLAN TO MAKING HEALTHY FOOD CHOICES

IN THIS CHAPTER I'll discuss with you the five Nutrition Success Principles we teach our personal training and nutrition clients. We use these principles with our clients to help them achieve dramatic results.

"One cannot think well, love well, sleep well, if one has not dined well."
– Virginia Woolf

Poor Nutrition Plans vs. Effective Nutrition Plans

How much better would life be if you discovered a diet plan that not only worked but that you could easily stick with?

Why is it so difficult to find a nutrition plan that works? With all the information at our finger tips, you'd think the "secret" diet plan would just be one Google search away. I guess too much information can be as bad as too little. Below find…

The Five Problems with Most Nutrition Plans

1. **Overly Complex** – We live in a busy world. While it will take some work and effort, many diet plans require hours of cooking and planning. They're just not realistic. Whether

it's weighing the food, excessive nutrient counting, or "carb cycling," you won't be able to maintain it. This is clearly a problem if you are on a quest for long-term health and fitness.

2. **Flawed Technology** – If I asked you to make ice cubes by boiling water, would you be able to? What if you tried really hard? Of course not. It's an ineffective technology. Many diets are no different. High carb/low fat diets pose some problems and they don't work for many people. And this brings me to problem #3.

3. **One Size Fits All** – Many "solutions" try to fit you into their box, which is backwards. The plan should fit to you. This is especially true when it comes to something as individualized as diet and nutrition. The truth is we all have unique likes and dislikes. What's more, everyone responds differently to different nutrients. While super low carb might be ideal for one person, it might leave another feeling drained and miserable.

4. **Too Boring** – I'm a firm believer that life is meant to be enjoyed. And this includes the simple pleasure of eating. It's sad that so many people miss out on this because of the belief that healthy and delicious are mutually exclusive when it comes to food. In addition, you'll never stick with something you don't enjoy. I mean, c'mon, how much grilled chicken can you eat before you feel like you're gonna grow feathers?

5. **No Accountability** – This is by far the biggest problem with most nutrition plans. Many of us fail to be consistent due to a lack of accountability. Once some solid systems to keep you on track are implemented, magic happens. We all need a little kick in the pants now and again and this is why simply following a diet from a sheet of paper doesn't work.

Now that we've covered the usual pitfalls of most nutrition plans, it's time to discuss the qualities of an effective program. Wouldn't it be great if you could finally get on a program that meets ALL of these criteria? Below I list…

The Five Qualities of an Effective Nutrition Plan

1. **Simple** – Anyone could follow it. Don't mistake this for easy. To achieve results that most people don't, you will need to do some things that most people won't (even though they're simple).

2. **Produces results** – Isn't that what you want, after all? To look and feel better? To experience positive physical change?

3. **Specific to you** – You can eat the foods you enjoy and do what works for your body type.

4. **Enjoyable** – You'll actually look forward to your meals. Whether you're at home, entertaining friends, or dining out, you'll have a plan that you like.

5. **Constantly motivated** – You'll have the support you need. Life can get tough and you need a support system to help you through the good and bad times.

TBBC's Nutrition Success Principles

Study after study shows that giving someone an exact diet plan doesn't work. There are a couple of reasons for this. For starters, these one-size-fits-all programs generally leave people more confused than ever. Our nutrition success principles are guidelines rather than an exact plan. This is because our lives are dynamic and our diet principles need to reflect that. Secondly, one-size-fits-all programs don't address the larger issue of why people fail on nutrition programs. While head knowledge is important, 80% of your results will come from behavior change, not new information. I'm going to share an inside secret that may damage some egos of personal trainers and nutritionists everywhere. This stuff isn't rocket science. The reality is if the average person followed the diet plan from a fitness magazine to the tee, they would probably get better results. Nobody does, though.

While there is no one-size-fits-all diet program that will work for everyone, there are some principles that are backed by research and produce great results in the real world. The following five guidelines are Total Body Boot Camp's Nutrition Success Principles. Are these the "be all end all"? Not necessarily, but let me illustrate how well they work. We recently started a nutrition accountability program called *Answers* where we coach our members to follow the guidelines. Here were the results.

*These are the actual numbers in **5 short weeks!** Nothing is changed to bloat the numbers.

Total participants – 11

Weight lost – 71 pounds

Inches lost – 15.75

Body fat lost – 19.08 percent

Wow! And these are regular folks just like you. Kids. Jobs. Mortgages. All the same stuff we all deal with.

There are no "secrets." It's really about just doing a little better each day. Which one of these guidelines do you think will make the biggest difference for you? When it comes to weight loss for busy people, these are your guidelines.

1. **Eat three regular-sized meals or eat a smaller meal every 3-4 hours** – I find that most people do better by eating smaller, more frequent meals. It helps keep the metabolism stoked as well as prevents overeating. As long as the rest of the "rules" are adhered to, go nuts and eat every couple of hours. With that said, we are all different and if the traditional "3 squares" works for you then go for it.

2. **Consume some high quality protein with each meal** – Some of my favorites are eggs, lean beef, chicken breast, and a high quality protein shake. If you think this list is booooooring, don't fret. There are plenty of options. How about

shrimp, salmon, mahi-mahi, or tuna? If you are a vegetarian, you still need to consume adequate protein. You'll just need to get complimentary proteins, which you can do with non-animal sources. An example of a complimentary protein is beans and rice.

3. **Consume fibrous veggies with each meal** – In addition to protein you'll need some vegetables with each meal. Instead of providing a list, just think about anything you'd put in a salad (not croutons or cheese!).

4. **Eat according to what you are doing** – Think of carbohydrates to your body like fuel is to your car. Recent research shows that carbohydrates (not fruits and veggies) are the main culprits of some terrible systemic issues like diabetes and heart disease. This is an individual thing and figuring out your carb tolerance can take some time and effort. Generally carbs are tolerated better after exercise so this might be a good time to enjoy some non-fruit/veggie carbohydrates.

5. **Maintain a balance of healthy fat in your nutrition plan** – Fat has been a very misconstrued nutrient in recent years. It may have even surpassed carbohydrates in the "misunderstood" category. There are three types of fat and you should eat a balance of all of them: saturated, monounsaturated, and polyunsaturated. Saturated fat generally comes from animal products. Monounsaturated fat comes from foods such as nuts and olives. For polyunsaturated fat, think flaxseed and fish oil. Believe it or not, consuming healthy fat can help you lose fat.

Now judging by these guidelines you can easily tell if your meal is an effective one or not. No protein in your meal? Doesn't qualify. It violates Success Principle 1. No veggies? As you can see that defies Success Principle 3.

Is this all the nutrition info you'll ever need to know? Probably not, but it's a good start. We're going to explore other topics but if you begin to feel overwhelmed, start with the above Success Principles.

Meet Heather

Heather is one of our awesome clients. She came to us at 30 years old and wasn't interested in making any dietary changes. She felt like that would be unrealistic since she worked two jobs, one in a restaurant/bar. She got some results by adding exercise 2-3 times per week to her schedule, but it wasn't enough to counteract the greasy bar food she was eating. She was still feeling sluggish and the pounds just weren't coming off.

I managed to convince her to give our Success Principles a shot. She was able to give up the wings and fries. Six weeks later she was down almost 20 pounds and in the best shape of her life. She followed the principles really well and was surprised how easy they were to actually follow.

Heather couldn't imagine herself not eating the bar food. Then she realized it was more about a change of mindset and she actually could change. It was nowhere near as hard as she thought it might be. Don't ever tell yourself absolutes about what you can or can't do. Where there is a will there's a way.

Hold Yourself Accountable

Now you know what guidelines to follow for an effective nutrition plan. But as I have said before, knowing and doing are two different things. We are going for behavioral change.

One of the reasons our Long Island boot camp members mentioned above did so well was because there was some built-in accountability. I love the quote, "What gets written down gets done." It's so true. If you want to make improvements in an area, you must put your attention there. You have to track what you want to improve. Here are two phenomenal ways to track yourself in regards to nutrition.

Basic journaling – Basic journaling is great if you're the type of person that gets all wound up about the numbers. Simply write down the following each day: Time of day, what you consumed, how much, and one sentence regarding how you did overall. For example, a meal entry might look like this: "7 a.m. – 3 eggs, 1 mini bagel, and banana. Good energy today. Feeling optimistic." With this method you can use a paper and pen (which is what I do) or just type it into your phone.

MyFitnessPal – Get the app and just track your total calories. Don't worry about the exercise stuff, just the total calories here. Here is the trick to losing weight. Take a week or two and find out your baseline amount of calories per day. Get the average by dividing the total number of days (e.g. 7 or 14 days) into the total calories (e.g. 14,000 or 28,000). If you lost weight or body fat, you are probably on the right track. If you stayed the same then this is the amount you need to maintain your weight. If you gained then you know what that means! Keep in mind the calorie deficit only needs to be slight. For example, 10% should do the trick. So if you are eating 2000 calories you'll drop down to 1800.

Have Others Hold You Accountable

Basic journaling and MyFitnessPal are great and necessary for holding yourself accountable. However, even better is to have others hold you accountable as well. I find accountability to be one of the most overlooked components to a fitness program. We all need a little help now and again. You can't always do it on your own. Here are some ideas on getting accountability.

- Hire a coach

- Tell people you trust about your goals and ask them to hold you accountable

- Share your goals on social media so you will be more likely to follow through

Meet Andy

When Andy came to me he was diabetic and overweight. He was frustrated that he was only in his early fifties but had to rely on diabetes medication. We put Andy on an exercise and nutrition regimen (with the consent of his doctor) to improve his glucose tolerance and help him shed some pounds. Here is an email he sent me after just a few weeks on one of our nutrition programs called "Answers."

> "I just wanted to thank you for your motivation, guidance, encouragement, and support with the answers group. I have lost a total of 23 pounds, which I am sure is actually more because I have gained muscle from my TBBC training and I feel great.
>
> "Most importantly I received my blood test results from my doctor and they came down so much in such a short period of time that my doctor said it was 'remarkable' how the numbers turned around for the positive.
>
> "I could not have accomplished this without your encouragement and of course your AWESOME Farmingdale team of Kathy, Bill & Sam.
>
> "Thank you again and I blame you for not having any clothes that fit. Thank goodness for smaller belts."

I love getting e-mails like that. It really motivates and inspires me to be able to play a role in such great transformations.

Enjoy Your Food

As you follow the five nutritional success guidelines, don't forget to enjoy your food!

I used to make the mistake of simply seeing eating as a necessity to endure, a way to get the fuel I needed. I now realize that eating and sitting around the table with my family is one of life's greatest blessings. I recommend you appreciate and enjoy your food. People are always on the go. Take a few minutes to slow down, enjoy your time, and connect.

I used to eat with my fork or spoon in my hand the entire time. I was basically just waiting to be finished. Now I try my best to put my fork or spoon down between bites. I don't want to be thinking about my next bite. I want to enjoy the current one. It's these little things people so often lose sight of.

Eating too fast can cause you to eat extra calories, up to 25 percent more! That's because your brain doesn't have time to signal to the body that you're full when you rush. Consider chewing slowly, taking pauses, and enjoying your food when you can. This can be quite challenging for some people. I challenge you to give it a try. Not only will you get more enjoyment, you'll be less likely to gain unwanted pounds, less likely to suffer from digestive problems, have a better bond with those you love, and have a better overall sense of well-being.

Food Lists

I know you might be wondering what foods might be included under the categories of lean proteins, fibrous veggies, starchy carbs, and healthy fats so I decided to provide you with lists. If you stick to foods on this list you'll be in good shape. Feel free to print out the list to keep with you as you shop.

Proteins

- Chicken breast (the real bird, not fast food meat!)

- Turkey breast (the real bird, not sliced lunch meat!)

- Game meats (venison, elk, etc.)

- Bison/buffalo (often leaner than regular beef)

- Very lean red meat such as top round and lean sirloin (grass fed is especially nutritious)

- Almost all types of fish

- Shellfish and other seafood

- Eggs

- Dairy products

Fibrous Veggies

- Broccoli
- Asparagus
- Spinach
- Brussels Sprouts
- Green Beans
- Bell Peppers
- Zucchini (summer squash)
- Lettuce and other salad greens (darker the better)
- Kale
- Cauliflower
- Cabbage
- Onions

Starchy Carbs – Again these are only if you can tolerate the carbs/calories.

- Sweet potatoes (or yams)
- White potatoes
- Brown rice
- Oatmeal (the natural, unsweetened kind!)
- Black-eyed peas
- Lentils
- Squash
- Peas
- Chickpeas
- Beans all kinds (black, pinto, navy, kidney, etc.)
- Quinoa (a natural whole grain)
- 100% whole grain bread and pasta products (use in moderation; even though they are made with the whole grain, they are lightly processed and calorie dense)

Healthy Fats

- Fatty fish (wild Alaskan salmon, sardines, mackerel, trout)

- Fish oil supplements

- Flaxseeds (ground)

- Flaxseed oil (as a supplement, not for cooking)

- Extra virgin olive oil

- Extra virgin coconut oil (for cooking; NOT hydrogenated varieties)

- Walnuts

- Almonds

- Other nuts

- Seeds

- Avocados

- Olives

- Coconut oil

- Natural peanut butter or nut butters (NOT the sugar-sweetened kind)

FREQUENTLY ASKED QUESTIONS

LET'S ADDRESS SOME common questions I get regarding nutrition. I wouldn't be surprised if you had the same or similar questions. By the way, the questions may be short, but some of my answers are long. Stick with me!

On the Road Again

Question: Hey Billy. I'm constantly on the road for business and I find it really difficult to stick with a nutrition plan. I'm either entertaining clients for dinner or grabbing fast food because it's convenient. Either way, I get frustrated not knowing which choices to make. How can I eat healthy when I'm on the road?

Answer: Some folks eat at restaurants because they enjoy it. Others eat out because they have no choice. I have a client named Bob who is a 58-year-old lawyer. Like you, he's often entertaining clients in the finest restaurants.

Many parents rely on restaurants as well. They might prefer a home-cooked meal, but if they are traveling for their kids competitions, they may have no choice.

Unfortunately, many times people wind up at restaurants when they are tired, hungry, stressed, anxious, and lonely. This can cause them to choose the most calorie dense foods (i.e. high sugar and high fat).

This is going to require a shift in mindset to be successful. It might sound overly simple but…be positive!

Remember that there are no "mess ups." There are simply opportunities to learn. If you can learn from an experience it is a success.

Now let's get to the eating on the road plan!

My first principle for eating on the road is *selecting healthful restaurant choices*. For instance, one time I was taking a friend to lunch. We were originally planning to go to a popular burger and beer joint. When we thought about how difficult it would be to eat healthy there, we decided on a different place.

Here are some things to consider when choosing a restaurant meal.

- **Check out the menu**. Do they only have fried foods or are there healthier choices as well? Do they allow special requests?

- **Choose your foods wisely**. Order foods that are baked, broiled, roasted, or steamed. Try to avoid anything fried.

- **Stick with lean protein**. Fish and low fat poultry are generally better choices than high fat options like cheese, sausage, and prime rib.

Let's move on to the second principle: *make better bad choices*.

When you are in a tough situation and there are no ideal choices, make the best of it. Here are some ways you can do that.

- **Remove the sour cream from the potato** – This greatly lowers the fat and calorie content.

- **Drain the dressing from the salad** – Dressings often carry many unnecessary calories. Most of the time we just need a little for taste.

- **Remove the skin from the chicken** – If you must get fried chicken, strip the skin off (especially if it's breaded) and only eat the meat.

- **Use portion control** – Eat until you are satisfied but not bloated.

The third principle is *to plan ahead*.

It's always going to be easier to make better choices when you plan ahead. You can plan ahead by…

- **Packing extra fruit with you**. Sometimes fruit is hard to come by when you're out and items like apples and raisins last a while.

- **If you are staying at a hotel, take a trip to the nearest grocery store**. This will save you time and money. You will also be much less tempted to call for room service!

- **Carry some carbs**. People usually overeat when they haven't been eating enough throughout the day. Bring some healthier options with you such as fresh fruit (oranges, pears, bananas), nuts, dry fruit, or veggie sticks.

Finally, pay special attention to dinner.

I mentioned earlier about Joe who I helped lose 10 pounds by simply reorganizing his meals. You might be able to do the same.

- **Put more emphasis on breakfast**. Breakfast truly is the most important meal of the day. It sets the tone for the day ahead. Eat some nutritious food like scrambled eggs or homemade pancakes and you won't feel the need to go nuts at night.

- **Refuel at dinner**. You don't have to starve yourself but the size of your dinner shouldn't be much larger (if at all) than breakfast or lunch.

If you stick to the program, you will see some very positive changes.

Busy Body

Question: Listen, I have 3 kids under the age of 4. I am just busy all the time. Do you have any tips for me?

Answer: I definitely hear you as I have 2 small children myself and I know how crazy things can get. There is hope! Here is what people need to know. 10 minutes of planning can save up to an hour later. Here's what some of my most successful clients do to make it work.

I call it my **3P Formula**.

P1 – Plan out your meals for the week. Scribble out what you will have each day for all of your meals and snacks. Ideally you will know on Sunday what you will be having for dinner on Wednesday. You can be flexible but get something on paper. Of course, then to make this work you have to buy all the ingredients you'll need to make the meals. This may seem like a lot of time and energy but it will make the rest of the week go so much smoother (and healthier).

P2 – Prepare the meals. Cook all the meals or at least enough for a few days in a batch. You might grill up a bunch of chicken breast or salmon, steam some veggies and rice, boil some potatoes, etc.

P3 – Pack the meals away. Put the meals in containers and store them in the fridge or freezer (depending on when you'll be eating them). Simply take them with you if you'll be on the road. You may even want to take a small cooler with you.

Just Beat It

Question: I'm a night owl. I love to watch Jimmy Fallon and other shows at night. They make me laugh. When I laugh, I snack. How do I beat late night snacking?

Answer: This is one of the most common problems I see. In fact, I also struggled with late night snacking for years. Know that you're not alone. The solution can be a bit complicated and take some time (and work) but here are some steps you can begin taking.

- **Identify the trigger**. What kicks the late night snacking cycle into gear? It might be cleaning up after dinner, flipping on the TV, etc. Write it down.

- **Identify the reason**. Perhaps you are bored. Maybe you think you need something sweet.

- **Identify the reward**. Maybe it's the sugar rush or the sound of the crunch from eating. Perhaps you think you deserve something sweet after a long day.

Realize that the trigger can't be changed. What can be changed is the actual habit (i.e. the late night snacking). Once you recognize the trigger, experiment with different habits. Perhaps you'll substitute the unhealthy snacking with something that's crunchy but healthy (e.g. carrots) or you'll take a walk around the block after dinner instead of snacking.

Are Carbs Bad?

Question: Should I avoid eating carbohydrates?

Answer: Carbohydrates are neck and neck with fats to win the award for the most misunderstood nutrient.

Here are some points to clear up the confusion regarding carbohydrates and fat.

- Everyone is different and needs a unique program.

- Stabilizing your blood sugar by limiting intake of refined carbohydrates will assist you in fat burning.

- While certain carbohydrates should probably be avoided, the following veggies contain phytochemicals and help prevent cancer: kale, broccoli, and cauliflower.

- If you tend to gain fat in the stomach area you may be more sensitive to carbohydrates. If you gain more in the hips then you may be able to tolerate them better.

- As a general rule, move more and eat according to what you're doing and you can't go wrong.

To answer the question, I'm not going to say that carbs are bad. Sure, I would avoid processed carbohydrates like cakes and cookies but fruits, vegetables, and whole grains (all carbs as well) can be very healthy. The key is choosing whole, fresh, minimally processed foods. You are much better off with potatoes than potato chips.

Everyone is different so I would suggest monitoring how you feel after eating certain carbohydrates (or any food). Do you feel satisfied and full of energy or bloated and in need of a nap?

Fat-Free

Question: I'm so confused about how to eat properly. I saw one book that claimed eating low fat was the healthiest way to eat and another that said that people need to eat fat if they want to burn fat. What gives? Is a low fat diet optimal for weight loss?

Answer: Yes, it can be very confusing. A lot of the "experts" can't seem to agree so how are people supposed to get this right? Hopefully I can clear up some of the confusion. Many people mistakenly believe they should avoid fat like the plague. Here are some of the benefits of fat that many people neglect to realize…

- **Protection for your cells** – Cells are what your body is made up of.

- **High energy** – While protein and carbs have 4 calories of energy per gram, fat has 9! That's more than double. What this means is that fat can be a very useful and efficient form of energy. You can use it for fuel!

- **Absorption of certain vitamins** – ADEK are fat soluble which means they need fat to be able to be dissolved.

Years ago it was reported that a diet high in fat was linked to some terrible things like heart disease. A funny thing happened though. As we started cutting down on fat, obesity levels (and heart disease) rose. We now know the true culprit was and is carbohydrates. I shouldn't blame excessive amounts of carbohydrates alone. The following factors are certainly not off the hook...

- Stress

- Smoking

- Excessive calories in general

- Inactivity

- Poor insulin sensitivity – This makes you much more likely to store the food you eat as fat

While I'm not telling you to make a complete overhaul on your diet, I will say that done properly it is perfectly safe and perhaps optimal for some to consume up to 35% of calories from fat.

*While all fats are a mixture of fats (saturated, monounsaturated, polyunsaturated), avoid trans- fat like the plague. No hydrogenated oils. Examples of foods that commonly contain trans-fat are cakes, pies, cookies, biscuits, breakfast sandwiches, margarine, crackers, buttered or flavored popcorn, doughnuts, fried fat foods, and frozen pizza. Here's a tip: if the food item can last in your pantry for weeks without getting stale, trans-fat may be responsible for keeping it fresh.

If you're not sure where to start, I think replacing carbohydrates with fats when you're going to be inactive might be a good place to start. Avocados are a great choice.

Case in point – I've been friends with Kathy for a while now. She started off as a training client, became a Director of First Impressions at Total Body, and is now a rock star coach. She helps many people transform their lives.

She's been in great shape for a while but in her words, she couldn't lose the last 5-7 pounds. She finally agreed to try manipulating her fats and carbohydrates with my help and BAM! Six short weeks later, she was down not only 5 but 10 pounds! She also experienced some other benefits...

- Better sleep

- More energy

- Improved complexion

- Better digestion – Turns out she doesn't digest certain grains very well and was experiencing some inflammation. Now that's a thing of the past.

Oh Snack Time. Oh Snack Time.

Question: I've tried other programs in the past that were so restrictive. Either I wasn't allowed to snack or I was only allowed something that didn't taste good. What foods can I have for snacks on this program?

Answer: Great question. Here is the short answer. If you follow the guidelines, you can snack on anything you see under the food lists.

With that said, healthy snacking can be tough. When people get tired, they tend to make poor choices about what they are snacking on. I recommend three things:

1. **Gradual change**. Don't try to change all of your eating at once. Start with just replacing one of your less than ideal snacks with a healthier option.

2. **Be mindful**. Many times we don't even realize what we are snacking on. We snack while driving. We snack while watching television. Keep in mind that those calories are getting digested whether we realize it or not. Make it a rule not to snack while you watch television or drive.

3. **Practice learning from your decisions.** You are not going to be perfect. We are all human and make mistakes. The key is to not beat ourselves up over our choices but to learn from them.

With that said, here's a step-by-step plan I recommend for Healthy Snacking:

1. **Clean out your cupboards**. If you're like most people, you will eat whatever is in the house if you are hungry enough. Will power is overrated. I find that the best way to avoid temptation is not to have it in the first place.

2. **Prepare**. Take 15-20 minutes before bed and plan out the next day. For example, put some nuts in a plastic bag and set a piece of fruit aside. You can make this planning part of your nighttime ritual.

3. **Keep your WHY front and center**. Things are much easier when they are fresh and exciting. It's when the daily grind kicks in that it becomes tough. Expect this to happen. When it does, think of the reasons WHY you committed to a healthier lifestyle.

4. **Commit to yourself and others**. Ask someone you trust to hold you accountable with the new behaviors you're working on.

5. **Beware of the enemy**. The enemy comes disguised in many forms. It might be the ad on the television. It might be your friend who tells you that "just one" won't hurt. It might be your own mind lying to you and telling you that you can't do it.

6. **Each week, improve more.** We should all constantly be improving. Ask yourself what you can do better each week. In an ideal world, what would your healthy snacking plan look like?

Here are some healthy snack ideas:

- Plain full fat yogurt – Optional: with fruit and/or nuts

- Cheese with fruit or veggies

- Hard-boiled egg with sea salt – Optional: with cucumber slices, avocado

- Nuts
- Nut butters (E.g. Almond, cashew, peanut) with raw veggies (carrots, celery) or sliced apple
- Dill pickles with cheddar cheese
- Avocado – Optional: with cucumber or tomato slices
- Smoothies – possible ingredients: yogurt, berries, nuts, flax seeds, avocado, coconut oil, coconut water, almond milk.
- Hummus and veggies
- Meats
- Spoonful of coconut oil with spoonful of nut butter
- Canned tuna and salmon – Ideally with homemade mayo. Add some chopped up veggies in a lettuce a wrap
- Kale chips - Remove leaves from stems and tear into small pieces. Drizzle in olive oil and sea salt and bake at 350 until edges are brown but not burnt for 10-15 mins. Deelish!

Know that you will not be perfect. Obstacles will come up. Changes will have to be made. Each week when you evaluate your habit, make changes accordingly.

Enjoy your healthy snacks. They are one of the great simple pleasures of life!

Cool Water

Question: I know it's important to drink a lot of water but I'm never sure how much to drink. How do I know if I'm drinking enough water and how much should I drink?

Answer: Drinking more water is one of the simplest things most people could do to improve their health so I'm glad you're asking. As a general rule, you should be drinking half your body weight in ounces. That means if you weigh 150 pounds, you should be drinking around 75 ounces.

As far as how you know, check the color of your urine. It should range from pale yellow to gold. Another general rule is that if you are thirsty, you've waited too long to drink.

Fluids should come from water, clear broth, and herb teas. Coffee (in moderation) also counts. This includes both decaf and caffeinated. Avoiding fruit juices would be a good idea, especially if you are looking to lose weight. This is because the sugar can prevent you from burning fat.

Action Step: Add one cup of water per day, perhaps upon waking.

Fluids help you feel full and will prevent overeating. I know I can be guilty of not drinking enough myself. I bought a huge water bottle that I take with me each day. This has helped a lot.

Carry a bottle with you and be sure to get at least 64 ounces in.

Just Add Supplements?

Question: I've seen some advertisements for supplements that can do anything from give me "6 pack" abs to make me look 20 years younger. I would love to believe these claims but figured I'd ask you before spending my money. Are there any supplements that actually help?

Answer: You're wise for being skeptical of the claims and asking. Quite honestly, most supplements are a complete waste of money. Oftentimes the best case scenario is a lack of results. You wind up with less money in your bank account and some wasted time. The worst case scenario is ending up very sick or even worse. Unfortunately many people have died as a result of taking a pill in search of physical improvement. This is serious stuff so I want to make sure you are well informed. My favorite professor in college, Dr. Lamonda, used to say, "Nothing will burn fat like physical exercise."

A bit more about supplements. Supplement sales in the United States are north of twenty billion dollars annually! Yes, you read that correctly. Twenty billion!

Many supplement companies prey on people who will do almost anything for a quick fix, especially when it comes to weight loss. Here are some tips to avoid falling victim to these types of supplement claims…

- **If it sounds too good to be true then it probably is**. Physical excellence takes time. If it were easy, everyone would be fit.

- **As my professor said, "Nothing burns fat like physical exercise**." The right amount of exercise at the right intensity is by far the best way to burn fat. And the best part is there are no negative side effects.

- **Think of supplements as a nutritional insurance policy, not a necessity.** A diet consisting of whole natural foods is superior to one consisting of many shakes and bars. Supplements can be used for convenience but they are exactly that, a supplement!

With all that said, I think a proper supplement plan has its place. It's all about taking the right supplements, though. There are several that have been proven to be beneficial. Personally, I keep my supplementation to a minimum. Below are the supplements I take as well as what I recommend my private clients consider and consult with their physician about.

Multi-vitamin/mineral formula – I often recommend a multi-vitamin/mineral formula as a first step in a nutrition plan. The reason for this is twofold. One, this is a great supplement to serve as an insurance policy. In an ideal world we are all getting the nutrients we need from food but as you know our world is less than ideal! The other reason is psychological. It helps you build a habit of taking care of yourself.

Whey Protein Powder – While I mentioned whole food being ideal, protein powder is derived from food sources. Protein powder can be a great addition if you aren't getting enough from food. It's also a great addition if you have the carbohydrate portion of a meal (e.g. oatmeal) but need a protein to complete the meal. Finally, some people have trouble ingesting enough food protein. In this case, a whey protein powder can be a useful supplement. I recommend you use the protein powder as your lean protein component portion of your meal. You want to make sure you are taking a high quality protein formula. Someone who is working out intensely on a regular basis is breaking down more muscle tissue and will therefore have greater protein needs. Most exercise enthusiasts will need somewhere between .8-1.2 grams of protein per pound of lean body weight. The good news is you don't really need to follow formulas. If you follow the Nutrition Success Principles outlined in this book, you will be getting the right amount of protein as well as other nutrients.

MRFs (meal replacement formulas) – Similar to the protein powder, the MRF would be used when actual food isn't available or convenient. These are great to bring on the road with you and use whenever you are in a pinch. Unlike protein powder, MRFs serve as a replacement for the whole meal. They contain protein but also carbs, fats, and other nutrients.

Fish oil – Fish oil is rich in DHA (this stands for a big word that's hard to pronounce) and EPA (another big word even harder to pronounce). These, as well as ALA (alpha-linolenic acid) are all considered omega-3 fatty acids. The benefits of fish oil are many, including…

- Cardiovascular function
- Immune health

- Increased metabolism
- Nervous system function

They also seem to be safe. Aim for 3-9 grams of total fish oil per day.

Green Powder – This is veggies and fruits that have been distilled and compacted into powder form. Green powder can function as a serving of vegetables and contain vitamins, minerals, fiber, and phytonutrients. Most people are simply not getting enough servings of veggies in their day.

Consuming fruits and veggies can reduce….

- Cardiovascular disease
- Certain cancers
- High cholesterol
- High blood pressure
- Type 2 diabetes
- Obesity
- Stroke
- Eye disease
- Asthma
- COPD (cardio obstructive pulmonary disorder)
- Osteoperosis

Another great benefit to vegetables and fruits (as well as a green powder) is that they counteract acid in the body and preserve bone and muscle.

Probiotic/Digestive Enzymes – 75 percent or more of your immune system is found in your digestive system. For that reason, you'll want to make sure your gut is healthy to help ensure optimal health. Making wise food choices and supplementing with both probiotics and digestive enzymes as a regular part of your program can provide some insurance that what you are putting in your body in terms of food will give you the maximum benefit and allow you to absorb all available nutrients. If your gut isn't happy, you won't be, either!

If you have any specific questions about nutrition or any supplements, e-mail me at billy@lifitnessbootcamp.com .

CONCLUDING NOTES

Some Extra Tips

SINCE ONE OF our values at our Long Island Boot Camp is Going the Extra Mile, here are some extra tips!

- Sometimes the best way to assess yourself is with the mirror

- Eating the right foods will boost your metabolism

- Increasing muscle will result in additional fat loss

- Eat slowly

- There are no magic pills or surgeries or injections

- You need to eat plenty of real whole foods

- Slimming spices – cinnamon stabilizes blood sugar levels, cayenne (hot sauces) boosts metabolic rate

- Green tea increases metabolic rate

- Avoid obesogens – These foreign chemicals can disrupt fat metabolism and lead to obesity. Some ways to avoid obesogens are to choose organic food whenever possible, avoid secondhand smoke and air pollution, and use glass rather than plastic when it comes to food storage.

- Poop once per day (I know that's gross)

- Drink plenty of water

- Get plenty of fiber

- LOVE your body!

Your Checklist

To sum things up, here is your checklist of things you need to do.

- Decide you are ready for a change and act on that. Do NOT wait. If you wait you may be setting yourself back 6 months or longer! There is never a perfect time. Act now!

Get some initial data so you know where you're starting from. This could be as simple as recording your body weight and taking a picture of yourself. You might also want to get a baseline for calorie consumption as mentioned in Chapter 9: *A Simple Plan to Making Healthy Food Choices.*

- Start tracking yourself by recording daily. Do NOT become obsessed with the scale weight. You just want to use it as a guide. Do the right things and the right things will happen.

- Shop for the healthy food on the lists provided so you can prepare some healthy meals.

- Get an accountability plan in place on your own or hire a coach.

Where Can You Go From Here?

I've dedicated my life to helping people transform their bodies and lives. I do this by helping them cut through all of the false information out there and offering the knowledge, action plan, and the accountability they need to succeed.

I love to meet with clients in what we call a "Success in Fitness" Strategy Session. I've got a great team of Body Transformation Specialists that I work with to help people just like you achieve the results they desire. Our clients even have fun while doing it! My offices are located on Long Island (Babylon and Farmingdale), New York. You can schedule an office visit if you want to make sure you get everything right. You can call our Babylon office at (631) 321-8222 or Farmingdale at (631) 225-7831.

Remember, wherever you are now in terms of your health and fitness, you can improve. Never forget that the choices you make each day will make you. Choose now to be an action taker. Decide on what it is you want to achieve and commit to it. Take some action each day that will lead you closer to your goal. If you do, you and those around you will be better for it. And you'll accomplish more than you dreamed was possible.

It might be hard to believe that this simple plan is all it takes to lose weight. I'm telling you it is. There is so much information out there that we tend to over-complicate things. Commit to these steps, follow through, and you will succeed.

Your health truly is your greatest wealth. I'm so thankful that you came into my life and me into yours. I'm so excited to see where our stories lead.

Made in the USA
Middletown, DE
21 July 2017